The Shift

The Shift

7 Powerful Mindset
Changes for Lasting
Weight Loss

Gary Foster, Ph.D.
Chief Scientific Officer, WW

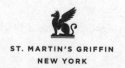

ST. MARTIN'S GRIFFIN
NEW YORK

Published in the United States by St. Martin's Griffin, an imprint of
St. Martin's Publishing Group

THE SHIFT. Copyright © 2021 by WW International, Inc. All rights
reserved. Printed in the United States of America. For information, address
St. Martin's Publishing Group, 120 Broadway, New York, NY 10271.

www.stmartins.com

Designed by Steven Seighman

Quiz items and score charts courtesy of Kelly D. Brownell,
The LEARN Program for Weight Control

Illustrations by Karolin Schnoor

The Library of Congress has cataloged the hardcover edition as follows:

Names: Foster, Gary D., 1959– author.
Title: The shift : 7 powerful mindset changes for lasting weight loss /
Gary Foster, Ph.D., Chief Scientific Officer, WW.
Description: First edition. | New York: St. Martin's Press, 2021. |
Includes bibliographical references.
Identifiers: LCCN 2021026565 | ISBN 9781250277756 (hardcover) |
ISBN 9781250277763 (ebook)
Subjects: LCSH: Weight loss. | Weight loss—Psychological aspects.
Classification: LCC RM222.2 .F6758 2021 | DDC 613.2/5—dc23
LC record available at https://lccn.loc.gov/2021026565

ISBN 978-1-250-88808-2 (trade paperback)

Our books may be purchased in bulk for promotional, educational, or
business use. Please contact your local bookseller or the Macmillan
Corporate and Premium Sales Department at 1-800-221-7945, extension
5442, or by email at MacmillanSpecialMarkets@macmillan.com.

First St. Martin's Griffin Edition: 2023

10 9 8 7 6 5 4 3 2 1

To my wife, Kathleen,
and our children, Katie, Ryan, and Kevin

CONTENTS

NOTE TO READERS

The names and identifying details of some individuals mentioned in this book have been changed to protect their privacy.

The approaches and techniques described in this book are not meant to be a substitute for professional medical or psychiatric treatment.

Reference to products, websites, and other potential sources of information does not mean that the publisher endorses such products or the information or recommendations in such sources.

The WW Logo is the registered trademark of WW International, Inc.

I'LL LOSE WEIGHT BY CHANGING THE WAY I ~~EAT~~ THINK

Shifting Your Mindset

This book is about losing weight and getting healthier, make no mistake. But it's not about what to eat. It's not a diet book. There are no recipes, no sample weeks of meals, no food recommendations or restrictions, no claims about which foods will make you gain fat or shed it. Does that surprise you? When people are on a weight-loss journey, their first consideration is usually something like, *What should I eat? What CAN I eat? Low-fat, high-fat, low-carb, high-protein, low-sodium, low-cal, high-fiber, Mediterranean, vegetarian, vegan, keto? Diet A or diet B? (Or diet C–Z?)* I've seen this whether at WW/Weight-Watchers, where I speak to members face to face or virtually at workshops around the country and the world, or among the thousands of people I have treated in group or individual settings, or among those I have just met who learn what my profession is. Everyone is focused on what and how to eat. I get questions like, *Can you really eat bacon and lose weight? Should I eat certain foods in combination? What's better, avocado or kale? What foods start my metabolism in the morning? What are the top five foods for weight loss? I heard about [fill-in latest fad diet]— what do you think?* People often want to be told what to eat.

Yet most people don't need me, or anyone, to script a meticulous moment-by-moment, meal-by-meal eating plan for them. When given a food choice (eat this or eat that), people generally know which is healthier. This banana (big, small, whatever) or that banana split? Deep-fried or baked? More times than not, it's clear. Sure, with a few foods, like dark chocolate or coconut oil, it's not quite so obvious how beneficial or not they are for our health. For the most part, though, we know.

NAME THE HEALTHIER FOOD[1]

1. (a) ground beef	(b) chicken breast
2. (a) whole wheat pasta	(b) white rice
3. (a) banana bread	(b) banana
4. (a) potato chips	(b) orange
5. (a) roasted potatoes	(b) french fries
6. (a) grilled fish	(b) fried fish
7. (a) half and half	(b) 2 percent milk
8. (a) oatmeal	(b) pancakes

---

1. (1) b, (2) a, (3) b, (4) b, (5) a, (6) a, (7) b, (8) a.

Despite this awareness, when people want to lose weight they focus on food, assuming there's something they haven't learned that an expert needs to tell them.

I get it. At the start of my career as a clinical health psychologist focused on obesity treatment, I assumed the same thing—food first, food last. But what I learned time and again through my work with my amazing patients was this: What you eat and how much, along with levels of activity, may seem to be all that count in weight loss, and they *do* count, of course—but without another crucial component, they will not add up to long-term weight-loss success.

That component is your mindset. How you think.

Look at mindset as having two parts: how you think about yourself and how you think about the journey you're on.

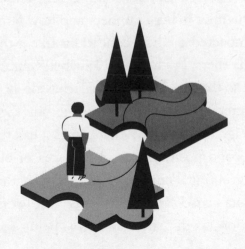

The ideal way to think about yourself is to accept you as you are now; a great way to do that is to practice self-compassion (the subject of chapter 1). The ideal way to think about the journey is to think realistically, flexibly, and with the big picture in mind; one way to do that is by identifying and countering unhelpful thoughts (the subject of chapter 2).

Let me share how I became convinced that mindset is critical for any successful weight-loss journey, and why, without the proper mindset, any success will be fleeting.

After majoring in psychology in college, I wanted to head straight to graduate school to become a practicing psychologist, but I wasn't 100 percent sure of my path. My advisor suggested that I first learn about the field, by doing research with psychologists. I looked for jobs at the University of Pennsylvania, in Philadelphia, about forty-five minutes from my home, and two positions caught my interest. The first was helping a researcher in family dynamics to better understand how family inter-actions impacted medical conditions like asthma, dia-betes, and others. I've had type 1 diabetes since I was six years old, so the idea intrigued me. But the job involved watching and coding videotapes of family therapy ses-sions for eight hours a day. That didn't speak to me.

The second position was in the area of obesity: A research group at Penn was focused on better under-standing its causes and treatments. The work caught my attention, as did the way it was being conducted.

Still, when I was offered the position with the obesity research group, I felt it was largely serendipity to find myself in that world. I had no previous interest in or meaningful knowledge of weight loss or obesity. I myself hadn't struggled with those issues. My mom was overweight but not in a way that made a great impact on me or, as far as I could tell, on her. Back then, the prevalence of obesity in the United States was roughly 15 percent, not the 42 percent it is today. I confess with some shame that when I started in the field, I, like so many, held a simplistic, frankly prejudiced view of people who struggled with weight. Concepts like "willpower" and "discipline" were never far from mind. I wince to think I could ever have harbored such a misguided, hurtful, scientifically insupportable view.

Fortunately, it was knocked out of me in a hurry.

My early work at Penn involved doing weigh-ins, evaluations, and interviews. I asked people about their eating and activity patterns. Our patients were bravely taking part in studies that evaluated a variety of ways—diet, medication, surgery, behavioral methods—to improve short- and long-term weight loss, as well as manage the multiple medical conditions associated with excess weight. One study measured the benefit of a low-cal diet versus an extremely low-cal diet; another, the Atkins diet versus a lower-fat diet; another, the effect of behavior modification versus medication versus a combination of both; and so on. My interest and passion in the field grew profoundly. Why? I realized how much I enjoyed helping people who were struggling with their weight. I admired their persistence, courage, and openness to change. At that point in my career, I was hopeful that some mix of diet, a certain type of physical activity, and behavioral techniques like goal-setting and self-monitoring could improve success, in the short and long term.

My understanding of the field grew with my one-on-one work at Penn, as well as my extensive reading of giants in the field, several of whom were right there on our faculty, and whom I was fortunate to converse with and learn from—in particular, Tom Wadden, Kelly Brownell, and the late Albert "Mickey" Stunkard. Tom and Kelly are psychologists; Mickey was a psychiatrist. They helped me begin to understand that things were not as simple as they appeared. I was captivated by everything from the emerging science around genetics and fat cells to the potential benefits of surgery to advances in behavior therapy to the impact of school environments on childhood obesity. I grew increasingly aware of the pervasive, persistent, pernicious weight-based discrimination and stigma that so many people experience. The book that affected me most deeply, both personally and professionally, was Mickey's *The Pain of Obesity*. In it, he describes, poignantly and painfully, the cultural norms that make us feel entitled to judge the (supposedly weak) character of those who have obesity. He provides examples of family, friends, health care providers, teachers, colleagues, strangers—all of us— propagating notions that are not merely untrue, but unjust and inhumane.[2]

During my time as a researcher, it became increasingly clear to me that those who were most successful at losing weight and keeping it off were not necessarily the ones who recorded every morsel they ate or movement they made, or who lost weight almost every week, or who attended every session or followed the plan perfectly. No, the indicator that most correlated with success was their perspective. Did they have their "head in the right place"? Did they have a "helpful mindset"? Did they think in a way that allowed them to deal with setbacks and "stay in the game"? When life got in the way, did they have strategies to help them cope and continue on the journey?

Mindset mattered, enormously. When people came back years later to check in with me, I saw it even more clearly: Those who had been the most successful had changed the way they thought, not just about the journey but about themselves. Yes, their eating and activity

---

2. In chapters 1 and 5, I will return to this important topic: confronting weight-based stigma and discrimination; the harmful, lasting effects they have on so many; and how individuals can better address it. This has long been, and remains to this day, the most meaningful part of my professional life.

had changed, but it was their mindset that made those changes stick.

I'd like to say it once more: Their mindset mattered. Mindset is the biggest influencer of our daily choices and our long-term success.

I got the sense that the work I was doing early in my career had the potential to change people's lives, and I was and am immensely grateful for that. My two most significant takeaways from that unique opportunity: 1) many people (as previously mentioned) have harsh, ill-informed views about those who live with overweight or obesity and 2) science-based approaches can make a very positive impact. Those two insights are why I've stayed in a field that I more or less happened upon accidentally some three decades ago. In the years since, I have published, with the help of many esteemed colleagues, more than 250 scientific papers on ways to better understand, prevent, and treat obesity.

The book in your hands, then, is not about what you eat but the thinking that influences what, how much, and when you eat. To reach your weight-loss goals, *what's in your head is just as important as what's on your plate*. When you learn how to manage your mindset, eating and activity become easier. When those happen, other elements of wellness often fall into place. Yes, the right mindset is critical for the weight-loss journey, but learning how to think about the journey and yourself pays dividends on other life journeys, too, like work or relationships. Its effects are profound and go well beyond what can be measured on a scale.

If changing your thinking sounds daunting, I hear you. We have so many thoughts a day—some estimates say 70,000, though the data to support that are sparse. A recent study using sophisticated methods for assessing brain activity suggests the number is just above 6,000 per day. Either way, that's a lot of thoughts! Words and sentences and images pop into your head as you go about your life, from an observation about your dog's sleeping position or how your left elbow feels slightly sore to a question about when your car is next due for service to a concern about your mother's schedule for the day—as well as thousands of other thoughts, trivial and consequential, brand-new and repetitious. It's like a rushing river—so how are you supposed to pause the flow long enough to be aware of the way you think, much less stop it or reroute it? On top of which, so many of your thoughts are automatic, coming without your even realizing it.

Let me assure you: You will not have to examine all your thoughts, or even most. Changing your thinking in the service of losing weight and improving your wellness does not require your whole life to be unpacked, reworked, and monitored. The simple, proven techniques in this book can help you tune in to your thoughts at select moments during your day or week and shift to a more helpful perspective. Once you get the hang of it, some days and even weeks will go by without your needing to focus intentionally on your thinking. That "new normal" mindset will become habitual. And that includes mindset shifts that effectively manage the single most common derailer of any weight-loss journey: setbacks.

A brief word about setbacks.

The vexing twists and turns of a journey happen to 100 percent of us, at some point along the way. Usually at many, many points. Progress in any area of life rarely, if ever, moves in a straight line. Have you ever lost the same amount of weight week after week after week? Do you eat the same things, in the same amount, every week? Come to think of it, have you been on *any* journey—wellness or life improvement or really *anything* with a significant goal—like that? None of us has. Setbacks happen. Maybe you gained a few pounds after a fun vacation. Or had a day where you ended up eating way more than you wanted. Or your weight loss stalled even though you ate precisely what you planned to that entire week. It happens.

Yet "diet mentality" is so often hostile to the presence and humanness of setbacks. Diet mentality is often characterized by—or not-so-subtly encourages—all-or-none thinking; an "I'm either dieting or I'm not dieting" worldview; dramatic and often unrealistic goals; and, perhaps most damaging of all, harsh treatment of yourself after a setback. That's why diets do not produce long-term change. They're only about what you eat. But success *also* needs to be about what you think. Changing those diet-based thinking styles to produce long-term change is a lot of what this book is about.

Here's the exciting upside to setbacks: If you can learn to manage them, then you're more than halfway to success. And *the skills in these pages become* more *powerful when you hit a snag.* They help you think in ways that get you back on track. You'll learn skills like recognizing an unhelpful thought and having an effective, at-the-ready counter for it, and developing awareness of your thinking style and altering thoughts that aren't serving you well. Armed with the research-backed, mindset-shifting skills in the following seven chapters, you'll know when your thinking is interfering with your progress and what to do about it, so it's working for you, not against you.

Some skills are repeated across the various mindset shifts described in the following chapters, though they're tailored to meet the individual problem explained in that chapter. You don't need to learn all of the skills in this book, or even most of them, to succeed. The select few that really speak to you should do it. You can master them so they become second nature and so that they help with more than just managing your weight. These mindset shifts can help lift your mood, make it easier to build toward any goal using small steps, focus on a more accurate picture of "reality," and provide non-eating ways to cope with emotions like stress, frustration, sadness, and boredom.

I'm not promising you perfection, some blissful, straight trajectory to your desired weight-loss goal. I'm not telling you "My way is the right way!" or "Nothing can stop you!" or any of the other cheerleading platitudes that characterize so many dubiously credible books and infomercials on weight loss. I can absolutely promise you meaningful progress if you follow the techniques in this book because they are based on extensive research.

The book is organized around seven mindset shifts. Chapter 1 covers the most fundamental shift of all: self-compassion. This is the cornerstone of a successful long-term journey; it enables and amplifies all the other shifts.

Chapter 2 covers the power of various unhelpful thinking styles to hinder progress, and how to counter them and develop more helpful ones.

Chapter 3 debunks the myth that large, dramatic goals are motivating and effective, and advocates instead for reasonable, specific goals that can be met, and fuel habit formation.

Chapter 4 describes the benefits of leveraging your strengths rather than trying to fix your weaknesses—a fundamental premise of positive psychology. Shifting to a strength-first mindset has powerful effects on how you view yourself and the journey.

Chapter 5 addresses body image, its determinants, and the pervasive weight- and shape-based stigma that so many people experience, and which plays a role in their (negative) body image. This chapter focuses on learning to value your body, as is.

Chapter 6 addresses how you can best obtain the support you need from others around you. There are no awards given for going it alone; you deserve to get the support you need.

Chapter 7 covers some of the determinants of happiness—perhaps unexpected—and the importance of the practice of gratitude in overall health and well-being.

Each chapter is grounded in science and my experience of over thirty years working in the field. As a psychologist focused on behavior change, I believe in the importance of not just what and why but, most importantly, how: how to get it done. How to make change happen. Therefore, each chapter ends with multiple techniques to help you shift your mindset. I have also included some valuable resources for each of the mindset themes.

Throughout the book are also sections called "My Shift," stories by people, in their own words, who made the shift.

In writing the book, I was also fortunate to sit down

for meaningful conversations with many of the world's leading researchers in approaches such as cognitive behavioral therapy (CBT) and positive psychology, and in areas such as goal setting, self-compassion, character strengths, body image, weight management, and more. These esteemed women and men have done pioneering research and clinical work, and I am grateful to include some of their insights in these pages.

Mindset matters. How you think is the key component to lasting weight loss. If your mindset is not working for you, then you'll want to shift it. In the following pages, you'll learn how.

I MUST BE ~~TOUGH ON~~ KIND TO MYSELF TO LOSE WEIGHT

Embracing Self-Compassion

"What's the single most important tool for success on the weight-loss journey?"

That's a question I often open with when I speak at WW workshops, in person or virtually. Then I look around the room—or at all my Zoom squares—and see people gathering their thoughts. Hands go up, members eager to share their answers.

"Persistence."

"Discipline."

"Willpower."

"Being active."

"Eating fruits and veggies."

Once everyone who wants to has spoken, I give my answer.

"Self-compassion," I say.

Since it's unexpected for many of them, even counter-intuitive, I elaborate.

"You're at the starting line of a journey. If part or most of your thinking is fueled by beliefs like 'I'm disgusting' or 'I have no willpower' or 'I can't believe I put myself in this position again' or 'I can't like myself until I lose weight,' do you think the journey will go well? Does that feel like a good starting place? That's YOU you're talking about! Are you feeling motivated, empowered, hopeful? How might it be different if you began the journey with self-compassion rather than self-criticism?"

They get it immediately. There's universal recognition—indeed relief—that there might actually be a better way than self-degradation.

Self-compassion. I imagine you intuitively know what it means. Being kind to yourself, especially when things aren't going the way you would like. Valuing yourself. Considering yourself worth taking care of. An outlook that frames things not as failures but as chances to learn and grow.

But self-compassion can be difficult to achieve—more so, on average, for those struggling with weight, because of the nasty characterizations that many people in our society make about weight. Many people think that being tough on themselves is the key to motivation, that the whole point of the journey is to *fix* flaws, and that when they lose weight, *then* they'll deserve kindness. I've heard it too often throughout my career. I vividly remember Katie, a happily married mom (kids aged ten and twelve) and lawyer in her early forties who wanted to lose fifty pounds. During our first two weeks together, she followed our behavior modification program at Penn meticulously, met her daily goals, and lost four pounds. While she had hoped to lose even more weight, she was pleased with her progress and herself.

Week 3, life got in the way. She was in the middle of a complex case, and her kids had a stomach bug. Katie ate more than she had planned—specifically, three slices of pizza one night and a midafternoon candy bar on another day. She gained a pound.

When she saw me, Katie's self-assessment was harsh and uncompromising. "This is terrible. I can't believe I did it again. I ate like a pig," she lamented. "Can you believe three slices? I'm a terrible role model for my kids. I know my husband is disgusted with me. I don't blame him."

The severity of her self-criticism was distressing not only to her but to me. I wondered how an extra slice of pizza could trigger such character assassination, leading her to question her suitability as parent and spouse. In practical terms, I wondered how she could find weight-loss success if each setback was followed by such a vicious self-attack.

Yet when I asked Katie to imagine sitting with a friend who had "messed up" the way she had, and if she would respond to her friend with the same vitriol she aimed at herself, she was quiet. She shook her head. "No, never," she said.

I hear the harsh statements that Katie and so many others make about and to themselves after suffering a setback in their journey.

I had two desserts yesterday. I'm weak.

I went off track again. I have no willpower.

Would you ever use this hopeless, discouraging tone on a friend who had just experienced a setback? Would you use it with any person you know? With a *stranger*? If your child used such language about a perceived failure of theirs, would you encourage that tone? Would you consider it productive?

So why do you talk like that to yourself?

When you experience a setback, imagine a friend describing it. "I can't believe it!" your friend says. "I followed the plan; I thought I was doing so well and the scale went up."

Now what would you tell that friend? Probably something encouraging like, "Don't be so hard on yourself. Think how much it would have gone up if you *didn't* do all that you did." Or, "Hey, you've been doing great! Look where you've come from. Hang in there!"

Note that encouragement does not mean lying. The things you told your friend are not made up or fantastical. You're not fudging facts. You're being encouraging and hopeful but also honest and direct. A good friend can be realistic and truthful while still being kind.

What if you simply extended the same courtesy to yourself that you would to a friend after a setback, particularly if your friend had just spoken unkindly about herself?

"Self-compassion is really just turning compassion inward," says Kristin Neff, Ph.D., one of the world's leading self-compassion researchers, codeveloper of the Mindful Self-Compassion training program, and a professor of educational psychology at the University of Texas, Austin. "If you think of what it feels like when you give compassion to a friend who's struggling, whether they're feeling bad about themselves or having some challenge in their life, we know what compassion looks like. We know how to use our tone of voice or body language. We know what to say to be supportive to someone who's suffering. Self-compassion is simply giving that same type of warm support and understanding to ourselves."

Extensive research shows that self-compassion "works" and can be applied to help those on a weight-loss and wellness journey. "Clinically, patients who do well over the long-term—four, five, ten years—are those who are basically able to put into practice self-compassion skills," says Gary Bennett, Ph.D., professor of psychology and neuroscience at Duke University and an expert in digital obesity treatments.

In the following pages, I define self-compassion in more detail and spell out its impressive benefits, prepare you for some weight-specific bumps, and, finally, share the evidence-backed techniques you can learn for a new way of thinking and being.

What Self-Compassion Is (and Is Not) and What It Does For You

There are three crucial components to self-compassion:

- being kind and understanding to yourself, rather than engaging in self-criticism, when you have setbacks or feel bad about yourself;
- mindfulness, or being aware of and accepting your experiences right now for what they are, without judgment; and
- common humanity, or recognizing that imperfection is human, that stumbling or not achieving a goal the first time (or fifth time) is something that happens to every single person, not just you.

Self-compassion is much deeper than self-like; it's a combination of self-understanding plus kindness. If you're self-compassionate, you don't blame yourself for that lousy day or beat yourself up over it. You might hate what's going on at the moment or how it feels like a struggle. But your core, your being, *you*: That's sacred. That's worth loving and protecting.

Self-compassion makes the wellness journey a positive process, not a punitive one. You're doing something for yourself, not against yourself.

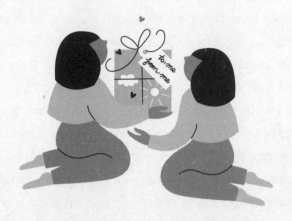

If your starting assumption is, *I'm worth taking care of*, you're in a position of strength. That's the point I always try to lead off with at those workshops. Strength leads to power. On the other hand, if you start from a position of self-loathing, you're at a disadvantage from the outset. You're starting with weakness rather than strength. Your attempt to make a positive change is pretty much dead on arrival. You're attacking your single most important ally, the one person whose support you simply can't succeed without. With self-compassion, you'll start stronger and stay stronger through the ups and downs.

Imagine something's gone amok in your journey. You had a setback. You followed your program and the number on the scale didn't move. You ate something unplanned. You got derailed. Now what?

Self-compassion works in these moments, helping you to accept what happened and hop right back on track. One study of women trying to lose weight showed the benefit of self-compassion: Participants in one group were each given a donut, then asked to do a self-compassion exercise, then given candy. Those in the control group were each given a donut, then candy—no self-compassion exercise in between. The women in the first group ate less candy than those in the second. One explanation? Those who focused on self-compassion made choices based on their intention that were healthier rather than spiraling into the self-critical thoughts that often lead to overeating. Another study divided soldiers on weight-loss plans into three groups: the control, a group that practiced mindfulness meditations, and a group that practiced self-compassion meditations. The self-compassion group lost more weight, on average, than the other two.

Research on weight loss tells us that those with higher degrees of self-compassion are better able to maintain a healthy eating pattern—likely because they're better able to handle negative feelings, forgive themselves, and move on when eating doesn't go the way they planned. But there are other wellness benefits that can't be measured on the scale:

- You're more likely to take care of your health (e.g., eat well, be active, take meds when recommended) even when you're ill, feeling low, or stressed.
- You're less stressed.
- You're motivated to be active for positive, internal reasons (e.g., it's fun, it makes you feel good) and not because you feel guilty or externally pressured.
- You're better able to let things go.
- You're less afraid of failure, hence you don't give up as easily or at all.
- You have a generally more positive outlook.
- You have a better sense of well-being.

An impressive list! Some of the people I've worked with over the years have pushed back, thinking that my suggestion to practice self-compassion is really a thinly veiled way to get them to view themselves unrealistically, as if they're perfect.

Not at all. Self-compassion does not mean that every little thing about you is awesome. You can value yourself while fully recognizing that you are flawed, like all of us, that there are things about you that you might like to change. Think of John Legend singing "love your perfect imperfections" in his hit, "All of Me." That's what you're saying: *I'm imperfect . . . and I still deserve kindness and love!* No matter what. If you're having a lousy day, you still care about yourself. In fact, you could be having a lousy day and not even *like* yourself very much in the moment—yet you still *care* about yourself. You're still kind to yourself because you know the lousy moment will pass, and *you* are not lousy. Self-compassion can help you see barriers more clearly so you can work to overcome them.

But wait (you might be saying): *If I'm trying to change myself, doesn't that mean there's something wrong with me?*

Again, no. A weight-loss or wellness journey is not about changing yourself. You are *not* your weight. You are not your body. The mindset-shift techniques in this book are designed to help you lose weight, get healthier, and feel better—*not* change who you are. You must already value who you are, your essence. You can be fond of the person you are while still aspiring to change and improve certain aspects; you want to move forward from where you are to where you want to be.

Self-improvement does not require self-loathing. What it *requires* is self-compassion. That's the fuel for your journey.

By thinking (or learning how to think), *I'm worth taking care of* or *I value myself,* you recognize that you're truly worthy of kindness and increase your chance for success in losing weight, attaining wellness, and changing other areas, too. Self-compassion is not mere pop psychology, feel-good thinking. Its effects are so broad and deep because once you learn to integrate it into your thinking, it changes what you *do*.

My Shift: Taylor

For most of my life I was a serial quitter. So I decided to take on the 52-hike challenge—do 52 hikes in a calendar year. It wasn't about weight loss; I just wanted to finish. The first time I tried the challenge, I got to 9 hikes before I quit. The next time, I made it to 36. In my third time trying, I finally completed all 52. But when I got to hike #52 and looked back on what I had accomplished, I realized I had done it with hate. I realized how horribly I talked to myself. The things my Inner Mean Girl was saying as I walked up the mountain—*You're too fat for this . . . You're not made for this . . . Everyone's passing you . . . You're so slow . . . You're never going to make it to the top.* The thing was, I was already on the trail! I was already heading up the mountain, doing this thing that's really hard! What good was it to tear myself down? None. I had "achieved" my 52-hike goal, but I could have enjoyed it so much more. I could have learned more.

I wondered: What would the journey have

looked like if I had been compassionate to myself the entire time?

I had completed something, so I thought, *What else can I not quit on?* I made it my personal development project to be self-compassionate, to pour more love into myself, to bring joy into the process. Sure, we're looking to get to the top of the mountain, literally and figuratively, but what is the experience of climbing it? How are you engaging with the people you're with? What are you learning every day? What is the journey itself like? I realized that before I started talking more compassionately to myself, I was losing sight of all the amazing things and magic that were happening while I was climbing and reaching my "goal."

With weight loss, I knew that recipes and types of food were important, of course, but I started to realize that mindset was key, and self-compassion was at the heart of it all. The key thing for me was consistency. That's what made it all click. Consistency compounds. It doesn't matter if I have one bad day or one bad week—all the good and all the intention add up over time. I learned to say to myself, *Look at what I'm capable of! This is just a baseline—now I know I can get here; let's see how much farther I can get.* I was eager to see myself stand back up after getting knocked down. I saw how being compassionate to myself made me stronger, able to show up for myself, able to come back and give my family and friends the best version of me. Why wouldn't I make that choice? To treat myself and talk to myself in that way, so that I could be the bold person I was meant to be?

Now I can rattle off in thirty seconds why I'm a badass, what I bring to the table for my career, my community, the world. It's a list I know by heart. And any time I slip into really negative self-talk, I tell myself—just like a good friend might—to be kind to myself and realistic. That's when I rattle off all the good stuff that I know is true about me.

Debunking Other Myths About Self-Compassion

Despite all of its benefits, many people I work with get tripped up by destructive myths about self-compassion. I'd like to address some of these mis-guided beliefs—beliefs that extensive research has already debunked—because they get in the way of a successful journey.

Belief: *Self-compassion just means making excuses and*

living in a fantasyland, allowing me to pretend that uncomfortable emotions, like sadness or loneliness, don't exist.

Reality: Self-compassion acknowledges that these emotions exist but recognizes them as part of being human. Even the happiest people don't feel happy all the time. What's important is that when you experience uncomfortable emotions, you show yourself kindness and patience. That helps you care about yourself enough to find activities that make you feel better.

Belief: *I am who I am. I come from a family of people who are hard on themselves.*

Reality: Actually, you can change. Some people naturally have more or less self-compassion, but it can be developed and improved through practice.

Belief: *Self-compassion is selfish because I've got other people I have to take care of.*

Reality: This myth can be particularly troubling for caregivers, who are predominantly women. Of *course* your life is busy, but there are techniques to cultivate self-compassion that require minimal time, and needn't even be practiced on a daily basis. Are you worth "putting first"? Although the analogy has been made many times, think of the flight attendant's pre-takeoff instructions to put on your own oxygen mask in case of emergency before helping a child or others in need. Laura, a WW member and mom of three from Indiana who eventually lost more than one hundred pounds after many attempts, says she only—finally—achieved success when she realized that "a healthier, happier, more present version of myself" was "the best gift I could have ever given my family and myself." We are, plainly and simply, more helpful and compassionate toward others when we're compassionate toward ourselves.

Weight Stigma and the Journey

Does this sound familiar?

The harsher I am with myself—and I deserve the harshness—the better I'll do.

Why do we say such things? What makes us think that that's an effective pep talk for losing weight or getting healthier or changing a habit? The myth that self-criticism is more effective than self-compassion—and make no mistake, it *is* a myth—is destructive. The myth assumes that the person you most need to believe in—you!—is a deficient person. A person you don't like or respect. "Teaming up" with such a person for self-compassion is like teaming up with the enemy!

Chances are, you didn't come up with the language you use to criticize yourself about your weight. It probably grew out of things said by others: family members, including parents; partners; doctors; strangers. It came from images on social media. It came from portrayals on TV sitcoms. Perhaps, in some way, it came from the relative *scarcity* of positive representations of people with larger bodies across all media (though, thankfully, that's changing). When I first started working with patients, I was shocked at how they echoed what they had heard from the world around them. They had experienced the harshness, internalized it, and turned it on themselves. And why not? Hear something enough—though it may be totally unfounded and mean—and you start to believe it. Decades later, unfortunately, I often still hear the same thing from WW members, patients, study participants, and many others about the toxic, weight-based messages they've been subjected to, including from the people who supposedly love them most.

Catherine shared her painful account of the day she went shopping for a wedding gown, found one she loved, stood excitedly before the mirror "in one of the rare moments I was not focused on my weight—and the owner of the bridal store said to my mom, 'You'll have to pay more because she needs the plus size.' It just knocked the air out of me. I was like, *Oh yeah, that's right, you're overweight.*"

Richie saw himself as a lesser, flawed individual for the most "logical" of reasons: because others did. "So many people in my life have said they don't like me and can't accept me at this weight," he told me, "and I know they're right."

And I have heard far too many accounts of people going for a flu shot or some other issue unrelated to weight, and their doctor makes a comment about their weight or blames their weight for whatever symptom they have, even if it's unrelated.

When you struggle with weight, you're often told outright or in subconscious ways that your weight signals a lack of character, a lack of discipline, or a fundamental weakness as a human being. The absorbed trauma can turn into negative self-talk. *I am despicable . . . I am unlovable . . . I have no willpower . . . I am lazy . . . Of course it's my fault . . . I'm a loser! . . . I have lived in a loose, indulgent, morally deficient way . . . I can't like myself at this weight . . . No one can like me at this weight . . . I must punish myself by following the harsh restrictions of dieter's prison.* And on and on and on. The more vicious, it seems, the better. You're determined to be hard on yourself because you think that's the ticket to success, the rough-but-galvanizing start that every journey needs. Yet in doing so, you deprive yourself of precisely the most vital fuel for success: yourself.

For perspective on just how wrong these messages are, let's apply this brutal, weight-specific mentality to an example that doesn't have to do with weight. If you had asthma, would you tell yourself, *I have asthma, so I'm a weak person?* No. It's a challenge; it needs to be dealt with; it doesn't mean you possess some central human flaw. It describes part of you, but it certainly doesn't define you.

In describing relationships, health, and other areas of

life, we commonly use words that convey self-kindness. When it comes to describing weight and body, though, much of that language is often nowhere to be heard.

The techniques later in this chapter aim to get you to look realistically at such messages as harmful (first those that come from the outside, then those that are internalized). Are the insults and critical talk even *close* to true? Are you a bad person because the scale went up by three pounds? Are you a bad, unlikable person, period? Of course not. Blaming yourself, blaming who you are as a person (or who, in that disappointed moment, you *think* you are as a person), is simply incorrect. Bogus. Eating is not a moral issue. Weight gain and weight loss are not moral issues. Your weight is not your worth. Your character can't be measured in M&M's eaten or not eaten.

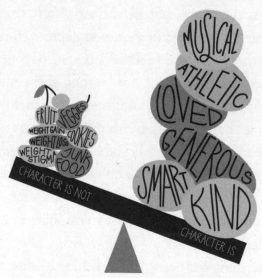

Perhaps nothing crystallizes internalized weight stigma as much as the routine use of the word "cheat" by those trying to lose weight. "I cheated today—I had a muffin I shouldn't have had." *Cheated?* When we say a student cheated on their test, we consider it a potential gateway to taking unethical shortcuts; when we say someone cheated on their taxes, it's pointing out a crime; when we say a spouse cheated, it's usually such an explosive event that it can put the marriage in jeopardy. How is eating a muffin on a level with these things? How can it possibly equate with making you an immoral or bad person?

The stigma around weight can deeply undermine the weight-loss journey. It makes individuals say irrational, untrue, and nasty things to themselves. You may be the CEO of a company, a marvelous artist or musician, a great parent, an incredible friend, and so on and so on—but when it comes to a weight and wellness journey, you have come to believe, *The more I hate myself, the better I'll do.*

Not long ago I had this exchange with Kevin, a patient: "I can't like myself until I lose weight," he said. "I'm despicable."

"You're *despicable?*" I asked.

"Well, I don't like the way I look."

"Okay. You're not loving how you look at the moment. Just so we have a fuller picture here, tell me about some of your favorite personal qualities."

After a brief pause, he said, "I'm a really good dad." After another pause, "I'm a very supportive colleague at work." A moment later, "I don't give up easily."

One conversation was not going to shift his entire perspective. But by continuing to look for what he valued about himself, a list that was surely numerous, obvious, and meaningful, he continued the momentum toward self-compassion. Once people express compassion about themselves, they're operating from a position of strength and are much likelier to sustain momentum. It's a positive loop.

If tough love (more like "vicious love," too often) worked with weight loss, I might suggest employing it. But it does not. The scientific data are clear: *When you beat yourself up, you are less likely to reach your goals.* There's no skill being developed, no concrete plan, no nourishing feedback loop.

That goes for non-weight-related areas, too. We see tough love routinely being dispensed in other dynamics—parenting, athletics, work. Except that, as stated above, research shows that tough love doesn't work. (There may be occasional exceptions, though not, it appears, with weight loss and wellness.) The fantasy that tough love leads to greater motivation, which leads to greater/quicker success, is just that: a fantasy.

Self-compassion is an idea you actively need to embrace. Not everyone knows naturally how to be self-compassionate. And in a society where people get blamed and stigmatized for their weight, when they're being told nasty things and being negatively stereotyped based on their weight, it's easy to see why so many believe the nonsense they've been told. They resort to self-criticism, feeling that that's the most effective way to stay "motivated" to lose weight.

And it simply is not. Approaching failure and difficulty with self-compassion actually *increases* the motivation to get up and try again, because you care about yourself and want to see yourself be happy.

I hope you feel persuaded enough to consider trying two techniques for building self-compassion. These skills are based on work done by top researchers and clinicians, including Drs. Kristin Neff, Christopher Germer, and others.

These exercises can be useful in the midst of a difficult situation or practiced at any time. Gradually integrate these techniques into your everyday life so they're available to you when the next challenge arises. It's not just the skill that's valuable, but your awareness that you possess such a skill to help power your journey. "Self-compassion is a superpower we have in our own back pocket, something we can use when we really need it to help ourselves," says Neff, "and we don't even know it's there."

You won't go from self-critical to self-compassionate

right away. It takes time to unwind habits formed over a lifetime. But just as you can change your eating and exercise habits, you can change your thinking habits, and self-compassion is a fundamental one. People who treat themselves with kindness, acceptance, and understanding—even if others sometimes do not—feel more empowered and confident about healthy eating and healthy activity, and about healthy living generally. I've seen this play out in the lives of patients, research participants, and WW members time and time again, with lasting results.

My Shift: Catherine

Whenever I started to lose weight, folks would say, "Oh, Catherine, you look good!" Or, "You're losing weight!" And my answer was always: "For now." Like I never believed it. Like, this is just what I do—put it on, take it off, put it on again, over and over. I had moments of success but I could never sustain the weight loss. I just couldn't understand why I couldn't keep at it. A piece of me started to think: *You're supposed to be this way. You're meant to be this way. This is your cross to bear.*

I didn't know my mindset was the real problem.

Around this time, I watched my young son, who had some developmental issues with his legs, go to physical therapy. I watched him teach himself to be patient.

Looking back, I realized that you can't be cruel to yourself and expect to stay motivated. I had to show myself some grace, the way my son had done for himself.

So the next attempt, I started to think, *Just hang in there.* That evolved into showing myself some grace. I didn't know that changing how I spoke to myself was going to change me. I remember stepping back and saying, *That's it. That's it! That's what you have to do for yourself! That's how you lose weight and keep it off. You do it by talking to yourself kindly and encouragingly and being aware of it.*

When I started to see some success and I recognized that I wasn't starving or having a bad headache all the time, I remember thinking, *Oh my gosh, I think I could lose weight and live this way.* That awareness and encouragement helped me.

That was in 2008. I didn't know it was about my mindset and being kind to myself. I have kept the weight off since.

If I had known this going into the journey

the first time—that it's not just about toughing it out—it would have made a difference. I would have been successful earlier. No one told me after a setback—and I certainly didn't tell myself—*Hey, it's okay. That ship has sailed. Let it go. It's all about the next step.*

But you need to love yourself like that, especially since people can be cruel.

SKILL BUILDING FOR SELF-COMPASSION: THE TECHNIQUES

Talk to Yourself Like a Friend

When you recognize how you show compassion to others, it can become easier to apply that compassion inward. When you have a setback or are otherwise struggling, use this technique to help shift the narrative and talk to yourself like you would your best friend.

1. IMAGINE IT'S NOT YOU BUT A CLOSE FRIEND who has had a setback or is having a tough time at the moment. What would you say to her/him? How

would you say it? Tone of voice is just as important as words.

2. **THINK ABOUT RIGHT NOW,** as you are in this moment
of setback or struggle. What are you saying to
yourself? What tone of voice are you using?
Does it feel cruel or kind? Speak the words aloud
or say them in your mind or write them down—
whatever works best for you.

3. **ASK YOURSELF IF THERE'S A DIFFERENCE BETWEEN YOUR
ANSWERS TO 1 AND 2.** If so, why? What might lead
you to treat yourself differently from others in
the same situation? What would change if you
talked to yourself the way you would a friend,
or the way a friend would talk to you?

4. **TALK TO YOURSELF LIKE A FRIEND.** This begins to shift
the narrative. The more you intentionally practice
this, the more natural it will become.

Note to Self

This exercise helps you to acknowledge and accept
what's going on with you, to talk to yourself with more
kindness, and to keep moving forward.

Grab a pen and paper, or open the Notes app on
your phone, and find a quiet place where you can write
uninterrupted for fifteen minutes.

1. **BEFORE WRITING, IDENTIFY SOMETHING ABOUT YOU THAT YOU'RE STRUGGLING WITH**—maybe a setback you have encountered or something that makes you feel like you're not good enough. Reflect on how it makes you feel: sad? embarrassed? angry?

2. **WRITE A LETTER TO YOURSELF.** Imagine you are a close friend or family member who loves and accepts you unconditionally. In your letter, express compassion, understanding, and acceptance for what you are struggling with. Consider the following as you write:

   • Setbacks happen to everyone—and it's normal to have things about yourself that you wish were different. Think about how many other people in the world are struggling with the same thing you're struggling with.

   • Recognize that setbacks are not your fault and that this "thing" may be the result of many factors.

   • In a compassionate, nonjudgmental way, ask yourself whether there are ways you could improve or better cope with the situation. Focus on how constructive changes could make you feel happier, healthier, or more fulfilled.

3. **PUT THE LETTER ASIDE** for a day or two. Set a prompt to reread it. Then, keep it close by for

the next time you have a setback or you're feeling down.

––––––––––– ADDITIONAL RESOURCES –––––––––––

- *The Mindful Self-Compassion Workbook: A Proven Way to Accept Yourself, Build Inner Strength, and Thrive* by Kristin Neff and Christopher Germer
- *Good Morning, I Love You: Mindfulness and Self-Compassion Practices to Rewire Your Brain for Calm, Clarity, and Joy* by Shauna Shapiro
- *Fierce Self-Compassion: How Women Can Harness Kindness to Speak Up, Claim Their Power, and Thrive* by Kristin Neff

What's Next

Self-compassion is the cornerstone of a successful journey; learning to replace self-critical thoughts with ones based on self-compassion has enormous benefits. It's key to manage self-critical thoughts because they get in the way of you feeling confident and inspired to reach your goals, and make it more challenging to overcome a setback.

Other types of thoughts that get in the way are less about how you view yourself and more about how you see the journey. Let's turn our attention to these in chapter 2.

I SEE SETBACKS AS ~~PROOF I'VE BLOWN IT~~ OPPORTUNITIES TO REFOCUS

Building Helpful Thinking Styles

Imagine you're a weather reporter in the TV studio. An ominous storm has started and you're describing it to your viewers. You're concerned about the storm's impact but can also see that it will blow over soon.

Now imagine you're a weather reporter on the ground, in the middle of the storm. You're soaking wet, nearly getting tossed around by the wind.

The job of both reporters is to describe the storm, but their experiences are quite different. The in-studio reporter has some distance from the storm, perhaps more perspective. The on-scene reporter is caught in it and can barely see what lies a few feet beyond.

Our thoughts are the storm. As the reporter on the ground, you get caught up in your thoughts, so it's difficult to see or do much else. As the reporter in the studio, you can observe your thoughts from a distance:

You can see the big picture and take actions that line up with your goals.

You want to be the weather reporter in the studio rather than the reporter in the midst of it.

Ellie, a patient of mine, was not yet the in-studio weather reporter. She and I had the following conversation, the broad strokes of which are similar to those I've had with many others over the years:

Me: "How was your week?"

Ellie: "Terrible. It was a disaster."

"What happened?"

"Saturday night I went to a wedding. I planned ahead, so I hadn't eaten anything beforehand. Then I got there and had a cocktail and appetizers. Actually, two cocktails. Usually I have one. I must have had eight hundred calories before dinner. You'd think that would have been a wakeup call. It wasn't. I not only had dinner, I had dessert. I totally blew it."

"Okay. So it sounds like Saturday didn't go as you planned. I hear you. Tell me about the other days."

"Oh, the other days, yeah. They were okay. I did my usual thing."

"What was that?"

"I did what I've been doing: planned breakfast ahead, same with lunch and dinner, and I had pre-planned dessert on Tuesday and Thursday. It worked out fine. I hit my calorie target every day."

"How about your activity?"

"Yep, I walked three times, like I planned. Each time was between twenty and thirty minutes."

The wedding "disaster" was one isolated event, yet I could understand why Ellie was focused on it. It felt so different from the other days, coloring her perception of the whole week. It was hard for her to put it in context—including the fact that in preparing for a big wedding meal, Ellie hadn't eaten for six hours, almost guaranteeing that she'd be ravenous by the time the trays of appetizers started making the rounds.

To her, it was as if she had driven over a road full of potholes, when in reality there had been one speed bump.

Regardless of what happened that Saturday evening, Ellie had been wildly successful the rest of the week, and it didn't happen by accident. To get three walks in, for example, she'd planned ahead, kept her walking shoes and other gear by the door, and left work on time those days. It was no miracle that it happened, and how it happened. She engineered it, each step of it.

"Okay, Ellie, let's just play this back," I said to her. "It sounds like for about nineteen or even twenty meals out of twenty-one this week, you did really well. Incredibly well, I would say. You did well because you had a plan and followed it. You hit your activity goals because you planned them and made them happen, each one. And yep, the wedding sounds like a tough night. You ate and drank more than usual. But even there, you planned for it, and then it backfired. So, really: You think the *whole* week was 'terrible'?"

Ellie's one-meal "disaster" did not upend her weight-loss journey; no one eating event (or two or three) ever can. But her unhelpful thought about it had the potential to derail her in a far more meaningful way. If that was her typical thinking "style" when a setback happened, and her response was persistently unrealistic, with a helping of unforgiving negativity, then the next time or the one after that she may just think, *What's the point? I give up.*

That kind of thinking is one of the biggest barriers to successful weight management. If you have an unhelpful thinking style (we all do, in certain situations), you will benefit from mindset-shifting skills that help you to recognize what's going on and then show you how to address it in a constructive way. Carol Dweck, Ph.D., the Stanford psychologist who helped to pioneer the area of mindset, defined two types: the "fixed" mindset, which assumes that our basic traits and skills are set, won't change much over time, and things are as they're destined to be; and the "growth" mindset, which sees setbacks as opportunities for growth and future development. The techniques in this chapter help you to shift your thinking style—your mindset—to better deal with setbacks.

Having unhelpful thoughts is not something deserving of blame. Our culture so often portrays excess weight in a harsh way, undermining your ability to have helpful thoughts about your weight (covered in some depth in the previous chapter). That societal nonsense is the perfect precursor for causing you to negatively overinterpret events, in a way that goes well beyond the facts. So when you face a setback—like Ellie's misbegotten wedding—it's easy to beat yourself up. And then to abandon the journey.

Unhelpful thoughts—all those that lead you to take actions that derail you—are nothing but "mind trash." The good news is that research shows that you can "rewire" your brain to adopt new, more helpful thoughts that give you power to act in ways that are productive for your journey. A key aspect of the various techniques in this chapter is pausing in the moment, finding a way to view your thoughts as objectively as possible, and if you have an unrealistic thought, countering it. By pausing, evaluating, and reacting, a powerful mindset shift can begin to happen. Such moments no longer derail your journey; they help propel you.

To readers who are thinking, *Sure, I recognize my unhelpful thought, but I deserve it. I did this to myself. I need to be even harder on myself*: Remember the need to be grounded in self-compassion. Without that, all the other good stuff can't happen.

Before I elaborate on the four main types of unhelpful thinking styles I've encountered, let's take a moment to delve into the connection between thoughts and actions.

Think . . . Do

What you think determines what you do. We know from cognitive behavioral psychology that what you think drives how you feel and what you do. Therefore, to do differently, you need to think differently.

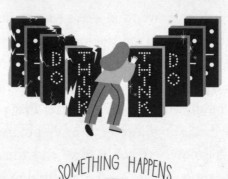

SOMETHING HAPPENS

This fundamental truth about human behavior—that thinking influences action—is scientifically proven, yet surprisingly many people don't recognize it. They more often believe that emotions drive actions, partly because feelings are easier to identify than thoughts, and that's profoundly true when it comes to weight management. People often don't even recognize their thoughts. If you're not aware of what you're thinking, how could you notice the impact it's having? Or maybe you are aware, but don't believe that your thinking style—the thought patterns, the types of thoughts you typically have—is the major obstacle to lasting success. If you think in unhelpful ways, your journey to long-term weight management will take the off-ramp over and over, regardless of how conscientious you are about what you eat.

It was in the late 1960s that psychologists first addressed weight management with behavioral treatment. Dr. Richard B. Stuart's groundbreaking work applied behavior analysis to the field. It attempted to reverse engineer the behavioral pattern: What were the antecedents of overeating? Its triggers? Its reinforcers? How did it happen? Under what conditions? This form of behavior therapy was expanded in the 1980s, exemplified by Dr. Kelly Brownell's LEARN program. The A in LEARN stood for "attitudes,"[3] and the program's inception marks the first time behavioral treatment included thoughts, in addition to behaviors, as something that could be altered to improve outcomes. This change was largely influenced by the pioneering work of Aaron T. Beck, M.D., in cognitive behavioral therapy (CBT). It didn't hurt that "Tim" Beck was on the sixth floor, and Kelly and the rest of us in Penn's Obesity Research Group on the fifth, but Beck's influence went well beyond that building. It profoundly changed the field of psychology and psychiatry, positively impacting millions, probably hundreds of millions, of lives since then.

Beck's premise and the foundation of CBT was

---

3. L stands for "lifestyle," E for "exercise," R for "relationships," N for "nutrition."

that the cause of unpleasant feelings and undesired actions was what people thought—their perceptions, the filters they used to interpret events. More than two thousand studies provided evidence that CBT helps people get better with various conditions, such as anxiety, depression, and sleep disorders. Just as important, studies showed that those who got "better" tended to stay better, since much of CBT is oriented toward relapse prevention. I won't outline a formal CBT program, but many of the techniques here draw from its insights. Current science-based approaches to weight management still use Stuart's behavioral techniques, such as self-monitoring and limiting cues and triggers, but also include CBT principles that focus on thinking habits as well as eating and activity habits.

"People's perceptions of situations influence their reactions," says Judith Beck, Ph.D., president of the nonprofit Beck Institute for Cognitive Behavior Therapy. "When people are in distress or engage in unhelpful behavior, some of their thoughts are distorted or unhelpful in some way. When they learn to identify and evaluate and respond to their thinking, then they generally have an improved reaction. We've seen that almost anyone can make short-term changes in their behavior, including their eating behavior. But to sustain long-term change, they really need to modify their beliefs, attitudes, and thoughts." With weight management, says

Beck, "a person sees the scale has gone up and thinks, *Oh, no, I thought I could do this, but obviously I can't. Nothing's working. I can't lose weight.* Many of these people with unhelpful thoughts just don't have the skills. No one ever taught them."

I want to refine something I said a few paragraphs earlier.

While it's true that if you change how you think, you change what you do, in truth it's a *three*-step process: If you change how you think, then you change how you *feel*, and then you change what you do. At times, when I've presented the dynamic this way to audiences around the country, I can see a look of fatigue set in. *Wait, I have to identify my thoughts AND my feelings?* Eyes glaze over. It's tempting to simplify the pivot to just thoughts → actions.

Make no mistake: Feelings are central. You behave a certain way because you feel a certain way. Put differently: Feelings are how thoughts influence behavior. It's crucial to understand that. When you get on the scale and see that you gained weight you didn't expect, you have thoughts that make you *feel* disappointed. It's that feeling of disappointment, of failing, that makes you take the action of stopping for ice cream on the way home. The anatomy of a setback begins with an unhelpful *thought* or series of thoughts (*I can't believe I ate those cookies . . . I can't do this . . . I might as well eat the rest of them since it doesn't matter anyway*) that give way to *feelings* (of despondency and futility) that drive the next *action* (quickly eating a bunch of cookies you didn't really want).

Is It Different When It's About Weight?

Human beings are not always consistent thinkers. Some people have one thinking style about one aspect of life—for example, resilient and open to compromise when it comes to, say, friendships or personal finances—and quite a different style when it comes to another aspect—say, about parenting or work life. On some issues or in some dynamics, a person's thinking might be reasonable; in others, perhaps extreme. True, some people have a thinking style that's consistent no matter the issue. But others default to one thinking style when it comes to weight, and *only* weight. Having worked with thousands of people over the years, I've encountered this phenomenon so often. If an issue is weight related, things are black and white, on or off. The same people who respond to setbacks at work or even at home with patience, moderation, and other helpful mindsets will respond to weight-related setbacks with unhelpful thoughts, such as, *I sabotaged myself on vacation, I'll never get this right, it's all my fault.* One patient, recounting a meal to me, said, "I absolutely blew it! What a complete, utter screwup.

I ate three thousand calories, I was supposed to eat twelve hundred, so I blew it, plain and simple. There's no other way to describe it and don't tell me there is. I'm done trying to lose weight." It's a good example of how thoughts lead to actions. The thought "I've blown it" can lead to the action of disengaging from the process altogether.

The good news is that there *is* another way to think about it, a way that's closer to the facts and far more realistic. Because thoughts—especially when fueled by an unhelpful thinking style—are not facts. They are simply things we say in our heads that we believe to be true.

To repeat: Thoughts are not facts.

When it comes to the weight and wellness journey, the ideal thinking style is this: realistic, flexible, and keeping the big picture in mind.

When you shift to a more helpful thinking style, you can achieve lasting success. Kathleen, a woman I worked with several years ago, moved in a social circle where thinness was overvalued to the point that it seemed almost required. It saddened me because she was a warm, accomplished, witty person, yet she couldn't see or feel that, because she had bought into her social group's belief that somehow she was "less than" based on her weight. It was as if her weight actually defined who she was as a person. It's one of the toughest things to witness as a clinician. That core belief impacted how Kathleen viewed herself and the journey. She was hard on herself and quick to make unrealistic assessments about any setback she experienced. She had a pattern of unhelpful thinking and lacked the tools to break out of it. As we worked together over the course of nearly a year, identifying and countering her unrealistic thinking styles and developing self-compassion, Kathleen started to chip away at her "negative filtering" (one unhelpful thinking style, as you'll soon see). She started losing weight, but she also began thinking in fresh ways. She found it liberating. I was thrilled for her and her growing sense of possibility that just maybe she could view the journey and herself more realistically and compassionately.

Five years go by.

As typically happens in research studies, participants are asked to return at some later point—one year, two, maybe five. This study had a particularly long follow-up of five years. We were seeing returning people one-on-one, assessing their metabolic rate, body composition, and mood, and then interviewing them about their overall experience. I remembered Kathleen well. We talked for a while. After I covered all the required research questions, I asked, "What was the best or worst part of the program?"

"Since I saw you five years ago," she said, "I've lost weight and regained some but kept in a healthy range. I've managed it. I feel good about that. But the thing that matters, that I'll always be grateful for, is what I learned about changing the way I think about the process and about myself. I'm not as harsh to myself. I'm more realistic in my thinking. When I have setbacks, I can see them in a balanced way. I can put them in perspective."

Kathleen and so many others taught me the most important lesson about these journeys: It's about mindset, and the ability to shift it to be both self-compassionate and realistic. It wasn't "just" about helping people lose weight, but helping them reach the goals that mattered to them. By shifting mindset, the courageous people I've worked with developed their very own power tool, one to be used when they wanted, in various areas of personal growth. A half decade had passed, and Kathleen didn't want to talk about how much weight she had lost (which is a fine thing to talk about, too) but how she learned a new way to think about herself.

Unhelpful Thinking Styles

Throughout my thirty years of experience in helping people manage their weight, I've noticed four styles that particularly get in the way of success:

- all-or-none
- negative filter
- once makes always
- don't worry, be happy

All-or-None

You're doing well: You stayed on track with your eating plan all week. Or you've gone to three yoga classes every week for a month.

Then you eat something unplanned. Or you miss your class.

Does this next thought seem familiar?

I ruined my whole day, you think after eating that unplanned something; feeling upset, defeated, hopeless, you proceed to eat more. (Why not, right? The day's totally wrecked.)

I've blown it. It's all over.

All-or-none thinking, as its name suggests, invites no middle ground. Things are either black or white, good or bad. If you're not perfect, then you're a failure.

You might relate to this kind of thinking because it comes naturally to many.

"All-or-nothing thinking comes up as an unhelpful thought pattern in virtually every area having to do with eating and weight," says Deborah Busis, Director of the Weight Management Program at the Beck Institute. "It's either 'I'm totally on my diet' or 'I'm totally off it.' Either 'I need to have zero sugar to lose weight' or, after falling off the wagon, the person eats way too much sugar. It's 'I really shouldn't have *any* carbs at all.' It can only be one way or the other." Categorizing foods as "good" or "bad" is a frequent manifestation of all-or-none thinking. It's one reason that a WW principle is that *all* foods are on the menu.

All-or-none thinking is extreme thinking—and the "none" part usually kicks in when there's been a setback.

I gained weight . . . it's no use.

I ate a donut . . . game over!

The reality, of course, is that the setback did *not* ruin everything. The focus should be on progress, not perfection—and progress is something best viewed over time, not in a snapshot. The key, says Busis, is for individuals thinking in this way to "catch themselves; if they make one mistake, don't let it spiral through the whole rest of the day, weekend, week, month, year. They need to view it as a mistake, not a catastrophe."

One way to recognize all-or-none thinking: how you go about setting goals. If an all-or-none thinker eats ice cream four times a week and decides that that needs to change, she or he might say, "I'm not going to eat ice cream anymore—period." This lifelong pleasure doesn't get whittled down to twice a week or even once—no, it's none, never again. But there's a greater likelihood of success if you set a goal that's incremental, not extreme. (I'll discuss this in detail in the next chapter.)

While all-or-none thinking can be common for those on a weight management journey, it can happen in other areas of life. If you forget to buy something at the supermarket, do you think, *The whole trip was a waste*, or if someone spills wine on the carpet, do you think the whole carpet is ruined?

Negative Filter

My goal of eating popcorn instead of cookies—I hit it only five days this week.

I lost three pounds this week but I'm still so far from my goal.

You focus on the one or two days, not the five or six. You take the negative, far less common event and make it the narrative.

When I've discussed this type of thinking with the people I've worked with who are trying to lose weight (like Ellie, at the start of this chapter), we talk about seeing the big picture and not depriving themselves of feeling success in the things that went well, not obsessing over the days they overate or didn't work out versus the days they met their goals. No one single eating event can disrupt their weight-control efforts. I say this not just to empathize with their current mindset (not that there's anything wrong with "just empathizing") but also because it's simple math: If 3,500 calories translates roughly to one pound, that means you would have to eat an "extra" 3,500 calories, with no compensating factors, for it to affect your weight . . . by one pound. So even one seemingly extreme, miss-the-mark episode is unlikely to affect your weight significantly, if you get right back on track. It's not that one eating episode that leads to weight gain; it's the unrealistic thoughts that lead to a series of unhealthy behaviors that lead to weight gain.

But even if that episode *did* make you gain weight: Is that all you should reflect on? No. It's certain that you did numerous things throughout the week to be proud of, things you can capitalize on to help get back on track. Zeroing in on that one unwanted eating episode is going to make you feel defeated and lead you to give up—and it simply doesn't reflect reality. It's a very selective, negative, self-compassion-free portrayal of reality.

Is this your thinking style with non-eating behavior? If on your performance evaluation at work you get mostly high scores and one mediocre one, do you tell yourself you're doing a lousy job? And that you're also a terrible person and you should probably resign? Suppose you looked at your relationships with the same mentality. Do you have a perfect marriage or relationship? Yet having a less than perfect one doesn't make us automatically think we're bad people, or unlovable, or don't deserve each other. Who has been a perfect parent? Yet being an imperfect parent doesn't usually make us think we're worthless, or that we should hand the job to someone else. We do a lot that's positive. Of course we want to be better, we'll try to be, and sometimes we'll even succeed. Often we won't. But we'll stick with the effort and give ourselves points for victories along the way.

The journey can be challenging enough. Robbing yourself of real victories is unfair to you, and unproductive. The next time you're feeling particularly upset or judgy about any one eating episode, missed workout, or blip on the scale, take a breath and see the big picture. A bump is a bump. It tells you nothing about the journey as a whole.

Once Makes Always

When I go out with my friends, I always drink too much and eat too much.

I gained weight this week. I'll never be successful.

The once-makes-always thinker builds permanent mountains out of episodic molehills. Since you acted a certain way in a certain situation, maybe more than once or twice, it's certain that you'll always act that way. These thoughts are often anchored by words like "always," "never," and "forever." Negative thoughts about one instance—along with a bit of selective history—are extrapolated, presuming a similarly negative outcome is preordained. Something "bad" happened? Guaranteed it'll happen again, and again, and again.

As with other unhelpful thinking styles, shifting away from this type of overgeneralization is, broadly speaking, about reframing. When working with people who tend toward once-makes-always, I aim to get them to see that the next instance doesn't have to be the same, each and every time—and in fact it's not a mystery how things turned out the way they did. There are usually clues. Ryan told me, "I'm never able to control myself when I go to a baseball game." I asked him to explain and he said that whenever he attends a game, he "always" has to have three beers, two hot dogs, and popcorn.

"Does that mean it has to be that way the next time?" I asked.

"It's always that way," he said, hopelessly.

We talked some more. What could he do differently? Could he order one hot dog first and then see if after a few innings he wanted another? Could he eat something before the game so he didn't arrive hungry? Could he focus on the food he enjoyed the most (hot dogs over popcorn)? Rather than think he had to cut out all beer, could he aim for two instead of three?

And what if Ryan didn't demonize his food consumption at baseball games, period? This kind of eating can be okay if limited to special occasions; if it has the effect of making Ryan feel stuffed and uncomfortable, say, then it's obviously worth changing.

As with other unhelpful thinking styles, the tendency is not exclusively reserved for eating behavior alone.

I felt awkward during that conversation . . . I'm always so awkward.

Another breakup. I'll never find love that will last.

He/She didn't call back. Nobody likes me.

Once, or even several times, does not equal always (or never). This type of overgeneralized forecasting drains fuel from the journey. If something didn't go as you wanted, think about how it happened and what you could do differently next time. (See chapter 3 for more on this.) Your new approach will keep you focused on actionable next steps rather than edicts about always or never, based on one or two examples.

Don't Worry, Be Happy

It's great during your weight-loss journey to show yourself compassion—it's more than great: It's a must for success. At times you need to give yourself slack. We all do. When things aren't going quite as you'd hoped, there's another key component for staying on track: your plan, and the more specific, the better. When people in our weight-management programs experienced backsliding, I would try to tease out how they were addressing it. "Things will be better next week," said Carole.

Me: "Great. Tell me how."

"I'll work harder."

"Okay, good. What's the plan?"

"I'll just be more focused next week."

Though you always want to begin with kindness toward yourself, the best thing you can do is focus on creating a plan and setting a doable goal for what's next. The person with a "Don't worry, be happy" thinking style is stymied not because of some deficit in personality or character or drive, but because of a simple lack of specifics.

"Don't worry, be happy" thinking points out, importantly, that unhelpful thinking styles will not shift in a meaningful way through mere positive thinking—or, perhaps more accurately, positive thinking alone will not help you achieve your goals. Many people believe that changing unhelpful thoughts is, at its heart, about having more positive thoughts. That's not exactly true. It's about swapping out unrealistic thinking for realistic thinking.

"Don't worry, be happy" can masquerade as self-compassion. You're not blaming yourself, nor should you, when you hit a setback. But the response can't begin and end with kindness toward yourself. It must ultimately focus on creating a plan and setting an action-ready goal for what to do next. You can't say things are going to be better and leave it at that. Nothing changes if nothing changes. Plans always work better than platitudes.

It Starts with Awareness

Imagine you're throwing a party and your very rude neighbor, who wasn't invited, walks in. You kick him out, but he comes back. You kick him out again, and he comes back again. You decide to stand guard at the door, but after fifteen minutes of this, you realize you're missing your own party. You abandon your post. At some point, Annoying Neighbor returns, only this time you decide to stop fighting it. You actually bring him a drink, then go visit with your friends across the room. Your neighbor hasn't become any less rude and annoying, but you accept his presence so you can enjoy the party. You stop putting energy into him, instead directing it toward what you can control and what's meaningful to you—talking and being with your friends.

Your thoughts are (sorry to say) the rude neighbor. Even if you're aware of them, it doesn't mean you like the thoughts or want to think them. By accepting that they exist, however, you're acknowledging them for what they are: thoughts, not facts. You're recognizing the situation and your thoughts without letting either take over or change your preferred route.

Starting to pay attention to and recognizing your thoughts—so many of which are automatic and have gone unnoticed for years—can be challenging. When you start to notice your inner dialogue, the volume, brutality, and unhelpfulness of your thoughts may surprise you. You may want to change the script overnight but shifting your mindset takes time. It takes time to turn healthy behaviors into healthy habits. Be patient with yourself as you explore your thoughts. Show yourself compassion. If an unhelpful thinking style was nourished over years, it will probably take some time to shift to a new, more helpful style. Kindness directed at yourself will help and ultimately speed the process.

Over the last forty years, numerous studies have been conducted on addressing and sidelining unhelpful thinking styles, by leveraging insights from CBT, Acceptance and Commitment Therapy, and positive psychology. Excitingly, the success enjoyed by participants shows that by following certain techniques, you really can shift your mindset to a more realistic one, giving you a new, powerful tool for achieving lasting weight loss. As you'll see, some of the following techniques are variations on a theme. You needn't master all of them, just the one or ones that feel most natural and doable.

My Shift: Matthew

My wife said she'd never met anybody as unkind to themselves as I was to me. I'd say unhelpful, cruel things to myself. I would slip up in a minor way, and find it difficult to have a day where I was just a little bit over. I was either wildly unhealthy and drank far too much and ate far too much cheesecake, or I was religious about everything that passed my lips. I was the master of catastrophizing. *Oh, well, I've gone over my goal for today, might as well just blow it all.* Or, *Oh, I've had a beer, I can't possibly go to the gym tonight because that would be really dangerous.*

I came to see my thoughts as triggers. Remember those "Choose Your Own Adventure" books? I'd have a glass of wine with lunch. Instead of saying, *That's it, I blew it, I'll start again on Monday,* I would pause and think, *Okay, a glass of wine at lunch—what does that mean? Does it mean I have to change my plans for the rest of the day, weekend, week? What were my plans for the rest of the day? Will that mean I go to the gym or that I won't go?* Those reality checks made me feel as if I was controlling the narrative rather than taking my unhelpful thoughts as fact or destiny.

SKILL BUILDING FOR HELPFUL THINKING STYLES: THE TECHNIQUES

Reality Check

When you identify unhelpful thoughts, Reality Checks enable you to shift to more helpful ones. These new thoughts can get you feeling and acting in ways that will aid you in reaching your goals. Use this technique the next time you hit a setback and feel discouraged, disappointed, or another emotion that has you wanting to make a choice that's not in line with your goals.

1. **I.D. AN UNHELPFUL THOUGHT.** Ask yourself, *What are my thoughts right now? What is the story I'm telling myself about this situation? What judgments have I made about this setback?* An example: After feeling stressed, you find yourself halfway through a pint of ice cream. You think, *I ruined all my hard work. I'll never get back on track. I should just give up now.*

2. **DO A REALITY CHECK.** Pretend you're a lawyer or a friend. As a lawyer, ask yourself, *Are there facts to back up my thought? What's the evidence to support it? What are the facts that prove this thought is not true?* For example, *Is it true that I ruined*

all my hard work? Is there really nothing I can do to get back on track? Is giving up the only thing I can do? Or ask yourself, *If a friend shared this thought, what would I say to her? How would I help him get back on track?*

3. **RESPOND TO YOUR REALITY CHECK WITH A NEW HELP-FUL THOUGHT.** Based on the answers to your reality check, is there another, more helpful way to think about the situation? For example, *Yes, I ate that ice cream without planning to. However, that doesn't discount all the progress I've made. It's just one moment and I can get back on track with my goals.* Or, *We all have times like that—it happens. Don't beat yourself up. You have what it takes to get back on track.* The more realistic your new thought, the more likely you'll respond to the situation in a way that gets you closer to your goals.

Noted, Accepted (and Then Take Action)

Sometimes we get hooked by our unhelpful thoughts: They're all we can see. By accepting your unhelpful thoughts and creating distance from them, you can recognize them for what they are—just words and phrases in your head, not facts. This can help you continue to move forward and make healthy choices.

1. **I.D. AN UNHELPFUL THOUGHT.** When you're feeling unhelpful emotions or responding to a setback in a way that will get you farther from your goals, ask yourself what thoughts might be causing this. What are the things you're saying to yourself?

2. **NAME THE THOUGHT,** as if you're observing it from afar. When the thought, *I'm never going to be able to do this* pops up again, say to yourself, *There's that thought again!* or *My mind is telling me that I'm never going to be able to do this. I often have this thought when I don't do what I'd planned.* This helps you to create distance from the thought, which in turn helps you to recognize that *you are not your thoughts.* It might help to imagine a cartoon character saying the thought, or to picture the thought as words on a page.

3. **COMMIT TO THE ACTION YOU WANT TO TAKE,** instead of the one that an unhelpful thought might lead you to. For example, you might think, *Just because I have the thought that I'm never going to be able to do this, it doesn't mean I have to throw in the towel. I can have that thought and still take steps toward my goals. I'll start tonight by cooking a healthy dinner for my family.*

Don't Worry—Make a Plan

When you reach a setback or challenge and have "don't worry, be happy" thoughts like *I'll deal with it tomorrow* or *It'll all work out in the long run* without also having a plan, it can turn a slip into a slide. Use this technique to keep treating yourself with compassion and understanding, while outlining specific steps to move forward towards your goals.

1. **TUNE IN.** Pay attention to the thoughts you have after a setback so you can begin to notice "don't worry, be happy" thoughts when they arise. Perhaps, for example, you were planning to start going to bed early but something got in the way of your doing so, and you thought, *Oops—guess I'll start tomorrow.*

2. **GET SPECIFIC.** Now ask yourself, *What specific steps do I need to take?* In the case above, you might set a bedtime alarm or plan to stop checking emails thirty minutes earlier to minimize distractions at bedtime.

3. **CREATE A PLAN.** Choose a doable solution, one you have confidence you can achieve, then enumerate the specific steps: Ask yourself what you'll do, when, and how you'll make it happen. For example, *Monday through Thursday at 9:30 P.M., I will shut off my computer, silence my phone, and*

open a book so I can wind down before it's time to go to sleep. (Monday through Thursday is better than *a few nights a week.* The more specific, the better.)

─────────── ADDITIONAL RESOURCES ───────────

- *Cognitive Behavior Therapy: Basics and Beyond,* (Third Edition) by Judith Beck
- *The Happiness Trap: How to Stop Struggling and Start Living: A Guide to ACT* by Russ Harris
- *Beck Diet Solution Weight Loss Workbook* by Judith Beck

| What's Next |

Now that you know how to shift unhelpful thoughts that might get in the way of your progress, you can learn how to set goals. Setting goals that are specific and reasonable is essential for short- and long-term success. It helps you to turn behaviors into habits. Chapter 3 shows you how.

I SHOULD TAKE ~~BIG~~ SMALL STEPS FOR BIG RESULTS

Setting Goals and Forming Habits

If you want a behavior to repeat, reinforce it.

That's the crux of psychologist B. F. Skinner's well-proven principle of positive reinforcement, sometimes called "operant conditioning." He showed it in his famous experiments with rats, pigeons, and people. It's the basis for hundreds of books for parents, teachers, and business leaders. The idea is pretty straightforward: behaviors that are reinforced will repeat; those that aren't, won't. Eating high-fat, high-sugar foods tastes good; they are reinforcing. Hitting the snooze button in the morning and turning over, rather than getting up early for a workout, feels quite good in the moment. The short-term reinforcing value of these behaviors makes them challenging to change, at first.

A less well-known but equally important concept of Skinner's is called "successive approximation." It builds the bridge from short-term to long-term change. In essence, it says: Reinforcement should not be contingent on achieving the "final" outcome. Completing any step in the desired direction of the goal is worthy of acknowledgment, even celebration. Thus, it's more effective to break big, longer-term goals into small, shorter-term ones—because all journeys need fuel to keep them going.

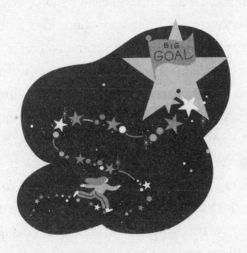

You deserve a reward for hitting a mark you set for yourself. If the goal you set is very high and far away, will there be enough interim rewards to reinforce that you're being successful and keep you going in the desired direction? You're likelier to have overall success by making smaller, incremental goals. As Gary Bennett, professor of psychology and neuroscience at Duke University, says succinctly, "People need some quick wins and early successes." So your journey is undeniably easier with smaller steps—both because you can reach your goal sooner and you go a shorter time before you get rewarded.

The shorter the distance between your current state and your desired goal, the likelier you are to succeed.

Say your goal was to forego the every-other-day 3 P.M. cookie and instead eat a banana at that time. When 3 P.M. Monday comes and you eat a banana, you feel good (reward) because you met your goal. You feel proud, a sense of accomplishment. You can also create a reward, like listening to a favorite song while you eat the banana. When you accomplish that goal, you're building agency. And when you eat a banana on Wednesday at 3, you're taking another step, building more agency. And so on and so on. You created a plan and with each and every action you're following the plan. You deserve to celebrate the steps, not just when you reach the final destination.

The key to the mindset shift in this chapter is this: You need to get your mind to a place where it says, *Small, specific changes are great.* Not okay. Not good.

Great.

Many people feel they must have "challenging" goals— that small goals are not as gratifying or engaging. They want to pursue a change only if it's "transformational." The idea of doing ten minutes of activity three days a week or having a banana instead of a cookie a few times a week won't cut it for them. They hear about modest, seemingly highly achievable goals and think, *Come on! What kind of a challenge is that?* They want to sweat. They want to moan and groan. No pain, no gain. If you're inclined that way and don't like that you eat ice cream, you might say, *Okay, I'd better throw out all the ice cream and never eat it ever again* (see "all-or-none" thinking in the previous chapter). Or you might decide, *I'm going to the gym five days a week, a minimum of forty-five minutes*—this from someone who may have been physically fairly inactive for some time.

People often think that this level of intense, transformative immersion is what's needed to fire them up, assuming that dramatic behavior change is what will lead to the dramatic result they seek. They're gunning for the finish line. They picture a future self who is excited, inspired, and energized about the eventual moment of achieving the big goal—not realizing that this initial ambitious push may create impossible standards that ultimately become roadblocks. It *lowers* the probability of success. This combination of dramatic goals, lack of success, disappointment, and disengagement creates what psychologists call the "action-intention gap"—the distance between what we intend to do and what we actually do. Setting small and specific goals and experiencing periodic success will fuel further behavior change and bridge the gap.

I don't mean to imply that you shouldn't dream big or that big dreamers can't have success. They can. It's the approach one takes to get to the finish line that has such a profound effect on the journey's success. The measured approach can and does work for the pursuit of transformational goals. A massive, dramatic, distant goal, while it may initially "startle" or shake you up, is usually doomed to fail unless you account for and develop the skills needed to get there—skillpower, not willpower. If you think that only the massive goals are worth pursuing, you're setting yourself up for setbacks that are avoidable; you may expect yourself to behave in unrealistically new ways that create friction with the rest of your life. Take the ice cream example from earlier. Are you really never going to eat ice cream ever again? That sounds improbable and not very enjoyable. And if and when you do eat it, you'll probably eat more than you want because you'll feel deprived and you had no plan to eat it—and now you have a setback on your hands. What if your goal was based on fitting ice cream into your eating pattern once a week? That sounds much more doable. You can "manage" that ice cream (i.e., how much of it you eat, that you're balancing it with a healthy dinner), no setback required.

When you fall short of a lone big goal, or any of the very big steps along the way, you'll believe you have failed. This is partly why mindset is important from the start: You want to pick goals that are short-term, specific, achievable, and relevant to you. All of that builds a feeling of success.

Big goals are not to be avoided. We have members whose goal is to lose a significant amount of weight—and they do. But having to take big steps to achieve them—leaping tall buildings—tends not to succeed. In my work over the years, I've seen so many people who embrace and thrive with the small-steps approach. It's transformational in helping to change the trajectory they were on. Smaller, daily choices have proved to be the far more reliable driver of dramatic behavior change.

As I wrote just a little while ago: The shorter the distance between your current state and your desired goal, the likelier you are to succeed.

That, in turn, fuels the journey.

The Power of How

How did it go well?

That's one of my favorite questions when I talk with people trying to make changes. When someone reports that they had a great week, I ask, "What went well? How did it go well? What did you do to make that happen? If it didn't go well, what could you do differently the next time?"

That's the crux of behavior change. If you can address those two questions—*If it went well, how did it go well?* and, *if it didn't go well, what could be done differently?*—

then you have an amazing gift: agency over the "how," over your next step, and, to a great extent, over the outcome you seek. Addressing the "how" shines a light on what's needed for meaningful behavior change and in a sense demystifies it: It's largely about setting doable goals and taking steps to achieve them—helpfully, at times, through the building of habits. When you get those right, you shift mindset; with this new positive, constructive, focused mindset, you're likelier to change those behaviors, build those habits, and reach those goals.

Of all the questions we ask, maybe none demand as much detail as those that pivot off the "how."

My patients and I do our best to leave no step undetailed. At the end of a session, I typically ask, "What are your goals for this week?"

"I want to eat better."

"What do you mean by 'eat better'?"

"I want to eat healthier."

"Okay. How do you plan to do that?"

"I want to eat more fruits and vegetables."

"What kind of fruits and vegetables? Let's pick a couple you like."

"Oranges and broccoli."

"Excellent. Okay, how many days a week do you want to do that?"

"Three."

"Good. Which days and what time of day? . . ."

At this point, the patient may think (and some even say), *Enough!*

Yet, tedious and annoying as it might sound, it's actually liberating. Thinking through the steps of "what" and "how" has the dual benefit of putting you in the driver's seat *and* generating a roadmap. It's one thing to know you want to drive to Texas; having the directions mapped out will help you actually get there.

And it works. Within a few sessions, the same people, when asked to state their weekly goals, will rattle off something like, "I'm going to do the stationary bike three mornings a week, Tuesday and Thursday at six thirty before work, Sunday morning at eight, for thirty minutes each . . ."

The beauty of going through this Q&A is the end product: You're left with a stripped-down, laser-like, highly specific goal. Not just the what (oranges and broccoli) but also the all-important how (all those details). If you say you're going to eat an orange three days a week (M, W, F at 3 P.M.), then it prompts the question: *How* will you make sure you have oranges in the house come Monday afternoon?

Blessed with an abundance of details, you're also able to assess the degree to which your plan worked. If the goal is as vaguely aspirational as "to eat healthier," then it's hard to evaluate if in fact that happened. You certainly ate healthily at many points during the week, but suppose at other points you ate something unplanned (almost a given, right?). How do you assess whether you achieved the rather broad "eat healthier" goal?

On the other hand, setting a specific goal helps you envision the steps you need to reach it, which better helps you achieve it (versus reflecting, after the fact, on why you didn't). If your goal is, *I'm going to walk three times, Tuesday, Thursday, and Saturday, around the field at my child's soccer practice, for fifteen minutes each*, you know if it happened or not, how many times, and if you hit your allotted fifteen minutes. If it happened, you know how—you wore your running shoes when driving your child to soccer practice; you brought your water; you had your podcast teed up. If it didn't happen, you know how—you were rushed getting out the door to soccer practice; you had too many texts to respond to by the time you got to the field.

The more you define *how* to navigate the road, the better.

Research has shown what factors help us set goals with success. At WW, we developed the four-step STAR principle:

- **S:** *Specific* goals (e.g., *I will go for a walk at 5:30 A.M. after brushing my teeth* or, *I will eat one banana with breakfast three days this week*). This is stripped down and laser-like, and gets at the what.
- **T:** *Truly doable goals*, to build a sense of competence and mastery, which builds self-efficacy,

which makes it likelier you'll keep up the behaviors to get there. We like doing things we're
good at!

- **A:** *Active* goals, focused on what you *will* do
instead of what you'll stop; this helps you get a
clear picture of what you're striving for (e.g., it's
easier to make your goal picking up the phone
and calling a friend when you're stressed than
planning to *not* eat when stressed). Being able to
envision the goal in action can help you identify
the steps needed to put the goal into action.

- **R:** *Relevant* goals. We humans have a need for
relevance, autonomy, and self-determination.
We prefer to engage in behaviors we choose and
that matter to us rather than those that others
think we should do.

Behaviors and Outcomes

Your longer-term goal, or North Star, is what you hope
to accomplish (e.g., *I want to lose x pounds* or *I want to
be kind(er) to myself*). That's your destination.

You set short-term, smaller, detailed goals to get
there (e.g., *I'm going to eat 1,300 calories a day* or *I'm going
to talk to myself as I would to a friend*). That's your path.

There's a distinction between what are called "outcome
goals" (*I want to lose fifty pounds* and *I want to be kind to*

myself are outcome goals) and "behavior goals" (*I will pre-plan three dinners a week* and *When I reach a setback, I will talk to myself the way I would to a friend* are behavior goals). My experience has shown me that it's best to focus on behavior goals—again, the shorter-term, the better. This needn't temper your ambition. You just want to avoid the derailing that so often comes when you shoot for the stars with no pit stops in between. Long-term goals are great, but without a series of short-term goals, they tend to be more aspirational than achievable.

Weight loss is an outcome goal, an amazing achievement, yet it's the result of a variety of short-term behavior goals. The goal to lose a certain number of pounds can be your destination, and yet if reaching this very tangible milestone is the main driver, the journey may be less successful than you hope. The more *behavior*-oriented your goals are along the way and the more you incorporate an action plan—the specific steps to reach those goals—the more likely you'll achieve the outcome you want. For that reason, I discourage my patients from setting weekly weight-loss goals. There are so many things that can affect weight in the short-term: humidity, body fluid shifts, sodium intake, time since you last ate. That's why changes in behavior don't always correlate in the short-term with changes in weight, leading to frustration and disappointment. I encourage people to focus instead on small, specific behavioral goals that they *can* control, and that will lead to their long-term weight-loss goal.

Studies have shown that choosing behavior goals rather than outcome goals translates to greater likelihood of success, because you are focused on things you have immediate control over (what you do) rather than things you have less control over (what happens as a result). "If you tell yourself, 'I want to be a healthier person' or 'I want to be a happier person' or 'I want to be financially comfortable when I retire,' you know those are really critical to you but you also need to articulate how you will get there," says Tom Wadden, Ph.D., clinical psychologist, professor of psychology at the University of Pennsylvania, and former director of the Center for Weight and Eating Disorders. "Setting realistic, attainable goals is critical—but it's really the action plan that lets you get to your goal. Goal-setting is one thing—that's great—but how do you get there, step-by-step?"

That's the S (specific), T (truly doable), and A (active) part of the STAR principle.

And there's that extra part about goals: Make sure they're truly your own. "Many people don't think through the behavior change they have to engage in to reach their goal," says Wadden. "They need to sit and really consider, *Do I really want to do it? Or do I feel like my spouse or my mom or dad or doctor wants me to, but I don't?*"

That's the R (relevance) in STAR.

If you can focus on what you want and what works

for you rather than on what others think you "should" do and on steps that are hard for you to take, then you will shift your mindset, which will help you make behavior change and help the journey succeed.

Aside from taking small steps, how can you make the journey easier, since behavior change can be challenging?

Habits.

Habits Make Things So Much Easier

We all develop habits without having set out to do so—for example, having a beer when you walk in the door after work or comparing yourself to each new person you meet. But a goal can lead to *intentional* habit formation, and healthy habits make your goals much more achievable.

A habit is a specific behavior formed when a specific cue leads you to do something, which is quickly followed by a positive impact; this "loop" is repeated enough times that the associations become nearly automatic. You now behave in this new way with minimal effort, consistently and over a long period of time.

Toothbrushing is the classic example. Once upon a time you brushed your teeth for the first time and everything about it was new, a laborious, time-consuming, conscious effort—not just the how of it

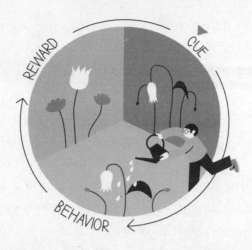

but the when and maybe even the why. (The where—over the bathroom sink—was probably taken care of from the start.) You likely argued with your parents about whether you had to do it or hoped they'd forget before they tucked you in. Soon enough, toothbrushing became an automatic impulse that, on cue—before you went to bed or soon after you woke up or after a meal—you knew, almost without thinking, to brush your teeth, engaging in this relatively effortless behavior. The positive impact or reward was *The toothpaste tastes good*, or *My teeth feel clean*, or *My parents are happy with me!*

Soon enough, habitual behavior no longer gets noticed: Think of how much concentration it takes when you're learning to drive, how much you have to think about the brake and the gas pedal and everything else . . . and when all those steps become "automated," you hardly even think of them once you get in the car.

While you drive, you're often thinking about other things. Often you arrive at your destination without much conscious effort because the cues of buckling the seatbelt, approaching an on-ramp, and many others trigger a series of automatic behaviors.

When a behavior is triggered and then reinforced, you're more likely to repeat it, which means it's easier to maintain, making it easier to become a habit. It doesn't feel like a struggle each time. You perform it in response to the trigger with little to no conscious thought, energy, or decision-making power. It just "happens." For better or worse, the behavior becomes entrenched.

Much of your day-to-day behavior is made up of performing predictable actions time and again under similar circumstances:

- putting your clothes in the hamper (or on the floor) when you take them off;
- sitting on a certain cushion on your couch;
- ordering popcorn when you go to the movies
- folding your towels a specific way;
- starting the coffee maker when you walk into the kitchen in the morning;
- crossing your legs when you sit down.

New behaviors can develop into habits over time. It's well documented—and your own experience probably corroborates this—that the process of turning a new behavior into a habit can be challenging. This is explained at least partly by how much of a continuing cognitive load—namely, thinking hard about what you have to do each time—is required to maintain a new behavior. Before this new behavior gets reinforced and possibly turns into a habit, how do you sustain it without burning out? By creating the scaffolding of small, doable steps.

Habits come in handy when we're stressed, tired, or otherwise taxed. It's in those moments that we have less capacity to make effortful, conscious decisions, so we're *more likely* to fall back on habits—and you want to make sure that those habits are ones that serve you well and are consistent with your goals.

Habits are a vital strategy for wellness. Research suggests that people who exercise at a consistent time of day tend to get more moderate-to-vigorous physical activity overall than those whose exercise routines happen at inconsistent times of day. Another study found that exercise happens more automatically for regular exercisers when they're cued by a specific location, such as running on a beach. Habit-development principles can also be used to help people sleep better. Creating consistent and predictable bedtime routines, for example, can improve sleep quality.

One of the truly powerful things about habits: Once they're established, *they're likely to continue even after a reduction in motivation, interest, or reward!* One study demonstrated that popcorn-eating moviegoers consumed as much week-old popcorn as fresh popcorn, despite stating that they didn't like stale popcorn. We do what we do. The mindset-shift techniques in this chapter help direct or redirect you to routinize the things that are beneficial for a healthy journey.

We tend to think of habits as observable behaviors—actions—but we also have habits of thought. *Ugh, I messed up again,* for example, or *I'm too out of shape to exercise.* Many of the techniques in this book (e.g., Reality Check, chapter 2) focus on monitoring and recognizing these unhelpful thinking habits so that they can be targeted and undone, edged out by new, more productive thinking habits. Developing helpful thinking habits and breaking unhelpful ones is vital. *Lasting* success is impossible without that.

How long does it take, generally, to develop a habit? The notion that a habit takes a set number of days to develop is a myth. While some say it takes twenty-one days to form a habit, evidence doesn't exist for this. It's believed that the idea stems from research in the 1950s that looked at how long it took plastic surgery patients, on average, to get used to their new features. That's it. In reality, there is no set time around habit formation. The time it takes to develop a habit depends on numerous factors, including the consistency of the cue, the complexity of the behavior, and the number of times it gets repeated in the same environment. True habits are slow to form, which is why starting with small, simple steps is often best. If you struggle to stick with new healthy behaviors, you're not alone. You're not weird or weak. It takes time. Remember self-compassion.

Skillpower Over Willpower

When embarking on a weight or wellness journey, so many people tell themselves, *This is all about willpower*. When their efforts falter, the most common responses are either to quit (*I just don't have enough willpower*) or to double down (*Guess I just need to have MORE willpower!*).

Realistic goal setting and healthy habit building are about skillpower, not willpower. You already *have* the will! Only the brave, the forward-looking, the determined embark on such life-transforming journeys. So don't beat yourself up or challenge your qualifications on willpower. The will is taken care of.

But willpower is unpredictable and not constant over time. When we decide to do something we'd prefer not to, or not do something we'd like to, we're exerting willpower. Willpower—invoking self-control or motivation—is essentially the opposite of relying on the habit loop. Willpower is conscious, effortful, intentional—and exhausting—whereas habits are automatic, occurring with little to no thought. Developing healthy habits, then, reduces your need to rely on willpower.

What you need are skills.

And what a great tradeoff that is, because willpower is frankly so often unreliable. Sometimes it works, sure. And often we must rely on it (for example, when you have to open your laptop to start working, or when you need finally to turn off the TV and head to bed). But the more decisions we make using willpower, the more each decision depletes our energy and renders it more difficult to continue making healthy choices. So when we're tired, stressed, or surrounded by lots of cues that pull us toward a choice that's not aligned with our goals . . . willpower is often nowhere to be found.

Studies show that those who consistently behave in "healthy" ways do so by relying on habits—skills—not willpower. That's because they don't spend lots of time deciding whether to make a healthy choice or struggling with urges that can pull them off track. They design their environments to trigger their habits. In other words, their surroundings reduce or eliminate the opportunity for unhealthy choices. Their daily routines are well-established—they more or less know what they're going to do and when—and they have to put little thought into it. Choices that might otherwise feel onerous (deciding what to eat, cooking dinner, getting out for a run, getting ready for bed on time) require little energy or thought. It has nothing to do with willpower. It wasn't because the sun, moon, and stars were aligned. The person succeeded because they created a plan and followed it. And then followed it over and over, until they were doing it almost automatically.

Building New Habits versus Breaking Old Ones

While the principles for both behavior changes—building up new, helpful ones and breaking free of old, harmful ones (perhaps by replacing them with helpful ones)—are the same, they'll probably feel different to you.

Creating a new habit is pretty straightforward:

- Identify a simple behavior to develop into a habit (e.g., meal prepping, stationary-bike workout).
- Pair it with a specific cue you'll be exposed to regularly (alarm, right after work).
- Make sure it's followed quickly, the sooner the better, by some kind of positive reward (a cappuccino, a hot shower, podcast while walking).
- Repeat, repeat, repeat!

Over time, the repetition becomes less thoughtful and more automatic: a habit.

Breaking an existing habit is a bit trickier. It requires an active disruption of the cue-behavior link. First, a relationship already exists between the cue and the behavior, and it's pretty strong. For example: when you're bored, you go straight for the TV remote; or if it's after 5 P.M. and you haven't yet planned a meal, you automatically order takeout for dinner. As long as that cue is regularly in your life, it's likely you'll repeat the behavior.

Identifying an old, not particularly constructive habit, one that's inching you farther away from what you're actually trying to do, is a great find, because you sort of "double" your impact when you turn it into a healthy habit. At 3 P.M., you tend to eat a chocolate chip cookie, in large part because they're always around. What if you had that banana at the 3 P.M. cue? Or suppose after putting the kids to bed—your opportunity to decompress—you find yourself on Instagram and eating a bowl of ice cream. What if you did that—except you ate a half bowl of fruit instead? Or what if you exchanged Instagram for a book? You want your replacement habit to have impact, and you also need it to be reasonable.

The exciting key to habit formation, be it forming new ones or breaking old ones, is that it powerfully increases your chance for success—*lasting* success.

My Shift: Jessica

When I started I was focused on the one hundred thirty pounds I needed to lose. It was daunting and I felt there was no way I could achieve it. So instead I focused on making small changes and short-term goals to help me get there. I celebrated every five pounds lost, no matter how long it took. I set goals I could control, like getting a certain number of workouts in each week. So even if the scale didn't go in the direction I wanted it to I could be proud of the choice I made that week. The journey's about so much more than a number on the scale. It's about forming new habits that will help me live the life I want to. And to create those habits, it takes setting small, realistic goals I can achieve and be proud of.

SKILL BUILDING FOR GOAL SETTING AND HABIT BUILDING: THE TECHNIQUES

STAR Power

You reach a big goal by setting smaller goals that "ladder up." Focusing on the task you need to do to reach your goal, rather than on just the goal itself, increases the likelihood you'll be successful. Follow the steps below to set a weekly behavioral goal using the STAR principle. Make it:

1. **SPECIFIC.** Start by being really clear on what you wish to do and the details of how you'll accomplish it. Want to eat healthier? Narrow that down to one thing you can do to eat healthier—for example, eating more fruits and vegetables. Then narrow it down further. Ask yourself what specifically you can do, when and where you'll do it, and with whom (if anyone). For example: *I am going to eat a salad with greens, apple slices, onions, and peppers for lunch at 12:30 P.M. on Monday, Wednesday, and Friday in my kitchen. I'll prep it after dinner the night before.*

2. **TRULY DOABLE.** When deciding what specifically you'll do, make sure you're realistic about what you can accomplish. If you don't have time this week to prep a salad three nights or you have many busy days running errands, then plan for one day. If you hate salad, try stir-fry. When you're set up for success, it's more likely you'll complete your goal.

3. **ACTIVE.** Once you have your goal in mind, make sure it's focused on doing something rather than stopping something. (*I want to eat a salad for*

lunch versus *I want to stop skipping lunch*.) This thought process helps you picture what you're trying to achieve.

4. **RELEVANT.** Make sure your goal feels meaningful to you. Goals should be about what you want, not what you think you should want. Does eating a salad with fruits and vegetables move you toward something larger that you truly want? Set behavior goals that are based on what you aim to achieve down the road *and* that will serve you in your day-to-day life.

Create a Habit Loop

At the foundation of every habit is the habit loop. Follow the steps below to create a loop for the habit you want to develop. Begin consciously to practice the habit loop you outline. The more often you practice it, the sooner it will become automatic.

1. **SELECT THE BEHAVIOR YOU WANT TO TURN INTO A HABIT.** Make sure it's one you can do often in the same context (i.e., same time, same place, etc.)—for example, making a healthy breakfast.

2. **ENSURE THE BEHAVIOR HAS A POSITIVE IMPACT.** You want the behavior to be reinforcing, pleasant, or something you'll be happy about when it's

accomplished. You can choose a behavior that's naturally reinforcing on its own, or build in a reinforcement. For example, if you want to turn healthy breakfast into a habit, choose to eat breakfast foods that you actually enjoy and look forward to, or add music to make food prep more fun.

3. **IDENTIFY A CUE.** Choose a cue that you come into contact with often—say, a certain time of day, in a recurring setting. The more specific the cue, the better—for example: When you press On for your morning coffee, you also start putting together your breakfast.

—————————— ADDITIONAL RESOURCES ——————————

- *Atomic Habits: An Easy & Proven Way to Build Good Habits & Break Bad Ones* by James Clear
- *The Power of Habit* by Charles Duhigg
- *Healthy through habit: Interventions for initiating & maintaining health behavior change* by Wendy Wood and David T. Neal (scholarly article)

What's Next

Reasonable and specific goals (goal-setting) in the context of cues and reinforcers (habits) will drive your long-term success. This mindset is quite different from lofty dramatic goals that rely on willpower. The next chapter shows you how to achieve another shift from focusing on weaknesses to leaning into your strengths.

Identifying your strengths and leveraging them can maximize the likelihood that you'll achieve your goals.

I NEED TO ~~FIX MY WEAKNESSES~~ ENHANCE MY BEST TRAITS

Leaning into Your Strengths

Sarah, a successful entrepreneur, spoke with well-earned pride about the ups and especially the downs she experienced while building her now popular and lucrative retail business. The near bankruptcies, the banks that denied her credit, the key employees who undermined her efforts, a recession: She persisted through it all. Her business eventually flourished. She was winning awards for her accomplishments.

When it came to weight control, though, even a mild setback threw her off balance. She saw each one as yet another sign that here was a goal that could not be reached, at least not by her. When I asked her to reflect on what qualities she used to navigate the uncertainty and difficulty of the business world, she said, without hesitation, "I believed in myself, I persevered, I never gave up hope, I could see the big picture." When I asked if she thought those qualities could help in weight management, she didn't answer. She got a faraway look, and you could see she was considering things. I could sense a reappraisal. It wasn't an earth-shattering revelation; she simply hadn't thought about it that way. Once she had, she became energized and confident, not deflated and demoralized. The beautiful part was seeing her realize that no "makeover project" was needed. In subsequent sessions as we continued to talk, she was increasingly able to leverage her personal strengths, especially perseverance and perspective, for her weight-loss journey. She began to focus and believe in her journey with an intensity I could imagine she had used to build a booming business. She had shifted to a new mindset.

It might not surprise you that most people who begin a weight-loss and wellness journey are focused at first on what they believe they need to change about themselves. *What's wrong with me?* they often think. *What do I need to fix?* There's a problem, to their mind, that needs solving. Our culture often highlights flaws and weaknesses and sees certain success (weight loss probably at the very top) as the elimination or diminishment of deficits, rather than the expression or building of assets. And it's not just our culture: Human beings often view their experiences through a negative lens. We can get stuck focusing on what we wish were different rather than on what's going well, on what we don't like instead of what we do. This also applies to how we think about ourselves. Our tendency to filter through a negative lens can get amplified when we face setbacks (see chapter 2). We can forget the numerous strengths we possess and get stuck on what we feel are our limitations. Then here comes the harsh voice insisting that *that*'s what's most true about us. In an effort to be more well-rounded, we attack our perceived weaknesses, focusing on those because we think they're the cause of our problems. We lean into those deficits, turning life into one big self-improvement project.

It's unfortunate that we so often "go negative" because, for one, it just doesn't feel great and, for another, research shows that it makes it tougher to address bumps in the road or to continue working toward goals. Since challenges will inevitably keep coming, it can resemble a game of Whac-A-Mole.

Part of what this book can do is help you to shift that mindset to a more realistic one—which, if you have an unhelpful thinking style, also means shifting to a more asset-based, not deficiency-based, mindset. So let's poke for a moment at the tendency we often have to take the fix-what's-wrong approach.

What if we didn't focus on weakness but (like Sarah, after some self-examination) on strength? What if, instead of emphasizing self-improvement, we emphasized self-celebration? To use a medical model: What if we focused not on disease but on health and wellness? It was just that type of thinking that, in the 1990s, launched the field of positive psychology, upon which many of the concepts in this book are based. While this approach does not deny the need to treat serious diseases such as multiple sclerosis, diabetes, or schizophrenia, it does posit—with the science to support it—that an asset/strength approach is more likely to optimize well-being. "Psychologists have learned over fifty years," wrote Drs. Martin E. P. Seligman and Mihaly Csikszentmihalyi, "that the disease model does not move psychology closer to the prevention of these serious problems. Indeed, the major strides in prevention have come largely from a perspective focused on systematically building competency, not on correcting weakness."

"We need negative experiences to learn from, motivate us, warn us, and help us grow," write Drs. Robert E. McGrath and Ryan M. Niemiec in *The Power of Character Strengths: Appreciate and Ignite Your Positive Personality*. "But those experiences should not define us. Reflecting on our strengths can help us offset those negative experiences, can help us figure out our natural best way to avoid them in the future, and can remind us that we have unique resources available to us in negative situations."

Success is not about fixing flaws, going from weakness to strength, but about leaning into strengths.

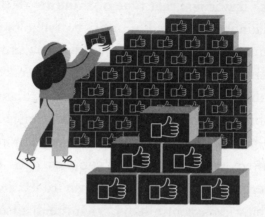

At WW, we meet people where they are, so they can find out what works for them. We don't want members to harshly restrict the foods they eat. The program takes an inclusive approach to food: Members are encouraged to think about delicious, healthy foods they can *increase* rather than focusing only on ones to limit. We reward all types of movement. We want members to zero in on the good, not merely because it feels better, but because it works better than the negative-leaning approach. Leading with your strengths—the qualities that come naturally to you and that help you feel like your best self—works. Positive psychology has shown it works. When you lead with your strengths rather than try to fix your weaknesses, you're more likely to make positive changes.

If you're struggling with weight loss or maintenance,

it's important to recognize that the many positive qualities you possess can be leveraged precisely for this sort of journey. Recognizing your personal strengths shifts your mindset toward capitalizing on what works for you and what you like about yourself. This helps you take steps toward your goals. It's positive reinforcement. When you focus on your strengths, you see yourself in a new light, build momentum, and respond to setbacks based on *what works for you*. You increase self-efficacy—your confidence in accomplishing something or developing a new skill. "When people learn of their core strengths, those strengths become psychological levers that they can grab onto for personal growth," says Neal Mayerson, Ph.D., clinical psychologist and a thought leader in positive psychology. "It's a paradigm shift from what's wrong to what's strong. People just feel more capable. They sit up straighter. They look you in the eye. Their voice becomes more alive. Because now they see possibilities, potential. Whereas before they were downtrodden with all the things that were wrong, and how they had to fix all that." Greater self-efficacy in weight loss–related goals (e.g., healthy eating, regular physical activity) is a well-documented predictor of success. The behavior of keeping at it (just putting one foot in front of the other and continuing, staying in the game): That's the cornerstone of long-term change.

In short, you can achieve your weight and wellness

goals without abandoning who you are; who you are at your best. If you do abandon who you are, in fact, any success is likely to be short-lived.

Can you easily name your greatest strengths? Many people can't because they're so focused on what needs to be fixed. Some may compartmentalize a strength, like Sarah, who could rattle off the traits that made her successful in retail but who needed a nudge to recognize that these strengths were equally available to her in other areas of life. I've worked with many people who have used a variety of skills to become successful in one area of life or another, and seemingly forget about those skills entirely when it comes to weight management. It's not that they're refraining from applying their strengths; often they're not even aware that they possess traits— kindness, prudence, forgiveness, perspective, courage, a host of others—that could be amazingly relevant and helpful to their weight-loss journey.

When people *do* recognize their strengths—and, intriguingly, simply recognizing your strengths can increase happiness—they can then apply them forcefully, making the journey easier. By intentionally employing strengths that come most naturally to you (and maybe even a couple of the more dormant ones you didn't know you possessed), you shift your mindset. You can increase your happiness for the longer term. Research shows that happier people make healthier choices.

What are the various strengths you might possess?

And once you know what they are, how do you deploy these superpowers?

Identifying Your Strengths

In positive psychology, lots of attention has gone into exploring character strengths. Many in the field see the benefit of getting people to identify their best assets, then applying those to an action plan that helps them achieve their goals more easily than with the "fix it" model.

We all want to know what makes us tick. Sometimes it can feel challenging to identify what comes most naturally to us, especially if we're used to focusing on what doesn't. You may struggle to identify your number one strength. You may struggle to find your top five. That's okay. Try visualizing a time when you felt at your best. What were you doing? Were there certain traits you were flexing? Does one strength come to mind? If not, don't fret. Know that we all have strengths, and many of them.

If you're having trouble spotting your own strengths, try doing so in your loved ones. It's often easier to recognize strengths in others. Once you've done that, *then* turn your eye inward. You may now find it easier to see what you couldn't before.

The most extensive taxonomy of character strengths

was created from a study led by Drs. Christopher Peterson and Martin Seligman, two of the founders of positive psychology, and conducted by fifty-five social scientists in the early 2000s. They sought to identify and classify "agreed-upon virtues" across cultures and generations. They studied world religions, philosophies, and assorted texts to identify the traits that make us human. After three years researching the matter, they came up with a list of twenty-four character strengths, across six broader virtues—courage, humanity, justice, temperance, transcendence, and wisdom—that are universal among humans. While there has been some discussion over the years over whether the strengths should be classified into six, five, or four groups of virtues, there has been little pushback on the strengths themselves.

According to their findings, we all have these twenty-four character strengths, the same twenty-four. Each and every one of us. (We may have other strengths, too, but according to their research, not universal ones.) We have them in different proportions, giving each human being a unique character-strength profile.

Take a look at each of the twenty-four strengths and their associated categories (from ViaCharacter .org/character-strengths) and see what resonates. Any sound like you?

COURAGE	**Bravery:** "I act on my convictions, and I face threats, challenges, difficulties, and pains, despite my doubts and fears." **Honesty:** "I am honest to myself and to others, I try to present myself and my reactions accurately to each person, and I take responsibility for my actions." **Perseverance:** "I persist toward my goals despite obstacles, discouragements, or disappointments." **Zest:** "I feel vital and full of energy, and I approach life feeling activated and enthusiastic."
HUMANITY	**Kindness:** "I am helpful and empathic and regularly do nice favors for others without expecting anything in return." **Love:** "I experience close, loving relationships that are characterized by giving and receiving love, warmth, and caring." **Social Intelligence:** "I am aware of and understand my feelings and thoughts, as well as the feelings of those around me."
JUSTICE	**Fairness:** "I treat everyone equally and fairly, and give everyone the same chance, applying the same rules to everyone." **Leadership:** "I take charge and guide groups to meaningful goals, and ensure good relations among group members." **Teamwork:** "I am a helpful and contributing group and team member, and feel responsible for helping the team reach its goals."

TEMPERANCE	**Forgiveness:** "I forgive others when they upset me and/or when they behave badly towards me, and I use that information in my future relations with them." **Humility:** "I see my strengths and talents but I am humble, not seeking to be the center of attention or to receive recognition." **Prudence:** "I act carefully and cautiously, looking to avoid unnecessary risks and planning with the future in mind." **Self-Regulation:** "I manage my feelings and actions and am disciplined and self-controlled."
TRANSCENDENCE	**Appreciation of Beauty & Excellence:** "I recognize, emotionally experience, and appreciate the beauty around me and the skill of others." **Gratitude:** "I am grateful for many things and I express that thankfulness to others." **Hope:** "I am realistic and also full of optimism about the future, believing in my actions and feeling confident things will turn out well." **Humor:** "I approach life playfully, making others laugh and finding humor in difficult and stressful times." **Spirituality:** "I feel spiritual and believe in a sense of purpose or meaning in my life, and I see my place in the grand scheme of the universe and find meaning in everyday life."

WISDOM	**Creativity:** "I am creative, conceptualizing something useful and coming up with ideas that result in something worthwhile."

Curiosity: "I seek out situations where I gain new experiences without getting in my own or other people's way."

Judgment: "I weigh all aspects objectively in making decisions, including arguments that are in conflict with my convictions."

Love of Learning: "I am motivated to acquire new levels of knowledge, or deepen my existing knowledge or skills in a significant way."

Perspective: "I give advice to others by considering different (and relevant) perspectives and using my own experiences and knowledge to clarify the big picture." |

This widely respected study led to the creation of the VIA Institute on Character's survey of character strengths, which has now been taken by over ten million people in nearly two hundred countries. The survey asks respondents to rate the extent to which they agree with statements such as

I experience deep emotions when I see beautiful things.

I always speak up in protest when I hear someone say mean things.

I am always coming up with new ways to do things.

I have many interests.

I always treat people fairly whether I like them or
not.

I do not want to see anyone suffer, even my worst
enemy.

From the responses, the survey generates a list of the
twenty-four character strengths, in order of the ones
you use the most. The top five ranked strengths are
your "signature strengths."

"We all have these twenty-four character strengths
but we discovered that certain ones are particularly
important to our self-concept and personal identity,"
says Mayerson, founder of the VIA Institute. "Once
you recognize that, you can come to understand how
your 'signature' strengths can be leveraged to engage
in any part of life—relationships, work, goal-setting,
whatever. Research supports that people who engage
more with their signature strengths in pursuit of their
goals are more successful."

In my experience, people who take the survey tend
to be unsurprised by their signature strengths. A typical reaction to the survey results and realizing one's
signature strengths is often something like, "Hmm,
yep, that makes sense." The quality feels innate. However, thinking of it as a strength often feels more

novel. In learning of her top strength on the survey, one woman noted, "Well, if you took that away from me, I wouldn't be me, but I never realized how much power it held!"

The most important reason to identify your strengths is to shift your thinking, from weakness first to strength first. Once you do that, you can focus on how to leverage that strength in your journey.

Putting Your Signature Strengths to Work

Your signature character strengths are the top five—the most abundant and available to you. Research shows that you can more easily improve your well-being by leveraging strengths that come most naturally to you, rather than trying to improve those that come less naturally.

If you don't wish to use the survey as an evaluation tool, Mayerson offers this thought experiment for figuring out your signature strengths: Imagine you're disallowed from using a small handful of the above twenty-four character strengths, ever again, for the rest of your life. Which ones would you most object to having taken from you?

Your signature strengths can theoretically change over time, but for many people they won't. Some who have taken the survey multiple times, across years, report that their top strengths rarely shift.

Sustained progress is more achievable when you apply your strengths. Suppose you want to start meal prepping. It takes time to do every Sunday morning, but you know it will set you up for success by ensuring you have healthy meals throughout the week. The prepping feels daunting. As soon as you start it, you become impatient. It takes longer than you want and you can think of a million things you'd rather be doing . . . so you focus on that. You start to try to become more patient. Likely you'll find it challenging to figure out how to "just be more patient"; that's never been you. Maybe you start feeling down on yourself, frustrated. You don't feel like you're moving the needle on your patience. It just doesn't work for you . . . but what if you recall your strength of being clever? How you always find solutions to problems and love solving puzzles? Now, you address meal prep as a puzzle. You focus on how to use your cleverness to make the activity more enjoyable. You turn it into a puzzle to solve. Likely, you'll find some solutions to make prep easier (for example, finding new techniques for packaging the food or cutting veggies that saves time). You'll feel proud of yourself and confident that you tackled something in a way that works for you.

What are ways you could apply *your* top strengths to *your* particular goals?

If perspective or kindness or forgiveness is near the top of your list, you might apply it to building self-compassion for when you have setbacks.

You can apply your signature strengths to help you set and reach food-related or activity goals. When you find ways to make eating healthier and being more active unique to you, it may become more natural. For example, if a top strength is

- *Love of learning*: research a new recipe for a healthy dinner; explore new methods of food preparation; find three foods or spices you've never tried before
- *Self-regulation*: keep track of what you're eating and review your progress for feedback on what to repeat or do differently next week
- *Creativity*: spice up healthy recipes in your own way; take pictures and make a Pinterest board / Instagram of the meals you cook
- *Humor*: listen to a comedian's podcast while lifting weights or going on a walk
- *Appreciation of beauty*: bike-ride, walk, or hike in nature
- *Curiosity*: read a book or watch a documentary while riding the stationary bike

Using One Strength to Help Another

As stated earlier, we all have so many strengths, many of which we're unaware. True, some we use more than others. Some are our go-to strengths when we're under stress. But they're all there. Maybe you turn your back on teamwork or judgment or spirituality, but that doesn't mean you can never access it, bolster it, and ultimately benefit from it at different points in your life, under different circumstances. Wherever your "lesser" strengths fall on your list, you can leverage each of them in a way that may help the weight-loss and wellness journey. An underused or dormant strength is not a weakness: It just needs to be awakened.

If you feel you need zest to be successful, then you can elevate it—strengthening a strength—by using one of your signature strengths. Take the example of Jim, who used to be known for his energy but was no longer that way. Every morning upon waking, the lethargy immediately set in. By around 3 P.M. every day, he was dozing off at his desk. "Zestful" was not a word anyone would attach to him anymore.

Was this lack of zest depriving Jim of all sorts of success, including weight loss? Was it even possible for Jim to live a zestful life again? Yes and yes. When he'd finally had enough, Jim decided to deploy one of his signature strengths—gratitude—to reinvigorate, or "tow forward," his dormant zestfulness. He started to focus on noticing and being thankful for the positive things he did feel, the things in life to be excited about. As his radar widened to look for things he was grateful for, Jim began to feel more eager for the day; to wake up with more energy, to feel more engaged in his relationships, his work, his daily activities, his whole life. He had more spring in his step. He was able to approach weight loss and wellness with much more enthusiasm, resolve, and confidence. On top of which: Employing a strength that hadn't been accessed in a long while is worth celebrating.

That's just one of many, many possible examples—and of course they don't need to impact just weight loss. I remember the story of Jane, whose kids were off to college and who had left her full-time job to freelance, and her once-busy, even chaotic, people-filled life had grown much quieter. Being around others and helping them had been one of her trademarks, bringing her and those around her pleasure and comfort. But that life was past, and it's not as if she could snap her fingers and make it, or that part of her personality that was so stimulated by it, just come back.

How did Jane rediscover it? She used another

trademark (and not-dormant) strength, humor, to tow forward her natural kindness and sense of teamwork. She rented comedies, watched comedians on YouTube, read books she once found funny, and listened to comedy albums. Slowly, she started feeling a bit lighter, day by day, a bit more eager to commune and laugh with others. She began sharing funny clips with her kids—something she could do in person when they were growing up (even if they didn't always find the same things funny). She watched lots of classic comedies, and found that the joy she got from them reignited her sense of being in the world and her need for people. She signed up as a reading volunteer, asked her closest friend if she would join her in starting a book club among their circle, and found herself getting outdoors more, especially on a local nature-preserve trail, where she was sure to interact with friendly, curious people. She was able again to share and help, something she had lost, and it was rekindled thanks to her enduring sense of humor and playfulness. Rather than feeling isolated, she was now engaged with others and felt more energized to take care of herself and her body.

Though it may not seem so at first, just about any strength (it's a strength, not a weakness!) can aid in your weight-loss and wellness journey—either by itself or by towing forward another waiting-to-be-deployed strength.

It's true that your signature strengths are easier to access and that you'll expend your energy more efficiently leveraging them. But committing to using a "lesser" strength can also help you on your journey.

SKILL BUILDING FOR ENHANCING STRENGTHS: THE TECHNIQUES

Mindset goes hand in hand with awareness—and you want to be more aware of your strengths. Once you identify your top ones, you can better leverage them to achieve your goals. These techniques help with identifying and deploying your strengths.

Identify Your Strengths

To leverage your strengths intentionally, you need to be aware of them. Use one of the following suggestions to identify which strengths come most naturally to you.

1. **EXPLORE WHAT MAKES YOU FEEL LIKE YOUR BEST SELF.** Ask yourself:
   a. At what time or during what activity do I feel like my best self?
   b. What makes me unique?

    c. What's one thing I would never want to change about myself?

    d. What comes most naturally to me?

2. **TAKE THE VIA INSTITUTE ON CHARACTER'S ASSESSMENT.** It is translated into more than one hundred languages (viacharacter.org/character-strengths). It will help you to identify which strengths you use most, but remember that all of them are potentially available to you.

3. **SPOT STRENGTHS IN LOVED ONES.** It's often easier to identify strengths in others than in ourselves. Think about your closest friends or family members or people you look up to. What strengths do you see in them? After you practice spotting their strengths, you may find it easier to turn it inward and recognize your own natural strengths.

Savor a Strength

This technique helps you remember your strengths so you can use them when working towards your goals and when you reach a setback.

1. **SELECT A STRENGTH YOU WANT TO LEAN ON MORE OFTEN.** If you're having trouble naming a strength, the previous technique can help with this!

2. **PICTURE TIMES WHEN YOU'VE USED THIS STRENGTH.**
   - What was I doing?
   - How did it feel?
   - What was the impact?

3. **DEVELOP A POSITIVE STATEMENT.** This will help remind you of your strength—for example, *I am strong*, *My humor is my greatest asset*, or *With my hopefulness, I can accomplish anything.*

4. **WRITE THE STATEMENT DOWN AND REFLECT ON IT OFTEN.** You might choose to say it aloud each morning, to remind yourself to lead with your strengths throughout the day. You might decide to think about it at certain key moments, such as before or after you step on the scale or after you've eaten more than you planned.

> ## Set a Goal with Your Strengths

Research shows that when we create goals with our top strengths in mind, we're more successful at reaching them. Why? When the steps we take to reach these goals line up with what makes us feel confident and like our "best self," we enjoy them more.

1. **LIST SOMETHING YOU'D LIKE TO ACCOMPLISH THIS WEEK THAT YOU MIGHT WANT TO SET A GOAL AROUND.**

For example: *I want more healthy options in my fridge and pantry when I snack.*

2. **BRAINSTORM HOW YOUR STRENGTHS MIGHT HELP YOU ACCOMPLISH THESE GOALS.** Have fun with this! For example, if your goal is to have popcorn and fruit available, and love is a strength, you could ask your partner or family to help with shopping or ask your kids to make a fruit salad with you as a Sunday ritual; if a strength is curiosity, grab a healthy food item from the grocery store that you've never tried before; if a strength is creativity, find a new way to combine foods or create a different method of preparation.

If your goal is to move more and a strength is leadership, share how you're moving with your community and invite others to join you; if a strength is adventurousness, take a bike ride to somewhere new; if a strength is bravery, try an activity you haven't done before.

If your goal is to shift to a more helpful mindset and your strength is gratitude, pause for a moment of gratitude every time you do something healthy for your body or mind; if a strength is kindness, try doing random acts of kindness for others, which can help you feel happier; if a strength is thoughtfulness, try journaling before bed.

3. **SELECT ONE OF THE IDEAS YOU BRAINSTORMED AND**

CREATE A SPECIFIC GOAL TO TRY IT THIS WEEK. Consider what exactly you're going to do, what strength you're going to leverage and how you'll use it, when and where you'll do it, and with whom (if anyone!) See chapter 3 for STAR goal-setting.

--- ADDITIONAL RESOURCES ---

- *Mindfulness and Character Strengths: A Practical Guide to Flourishing* by Ryan M. Niemiec
- *The Power of Character Strengths: Appreciate and Ignite Your Positive Personality* by Ryan M. Niemiec and Robert E. McGrath
- TED Talk: Shane Lopez, "Focusing on Your Strengths"

What's Next

Recognizing and leveraging your strengths rather than focusing on what needs to be fixed helps fuel the journey. Despite all that our bodies do for us, many people focus on what they don't like about their bodies.

It's such a common tendency that scientists call it "normative discontent," especially prevalent among women. Getting right with your body has many benefits both on and off the scale. The next chapter shows you how to shift toward appreciating your body, and away from equating your weight and shape with your self-worth. You will learn to value your body for how it is now and what it does to propel you forward.

I HAVE TO ~~HATE~~ APPRECIATE MY BODY TO LOSE WEIGHT

Valuing Your Body

When Ava went to a gathering or the town pool (or more likely *didn't* go to the pool), all she could think about was her body and how it looked. It was how she saw herself. It was how she believed others saw her— never mind that almost everyone, regardless of size, is much more concerned with their own appearance. She couldn't help but scrutinize the body parts of others that she particularly disliked in herself (neck, arms, thighs, belly); she lost every comparison. She wouldn't even think to dress in a fun, fashionable way, none of the pinks and turquoises and oranges and other bright floral shades she loved. "I can't wear something colorful," she told me, as if it was actually forbidden. "I don't want to bring any attention to myself." She believed she didn't deserve to dress in any way that aimed for attractive, so she gravitated to attention-deflecting drab colors, usually beige, or wore black for its magical "thinning" powers. She avoided the new styles that excited her, sticking with frumpy, which was not at all who she really was. It was all based on how central her weight and shape were to her self-evaluation.

Her negative body image had also put her life on hold, quite literally. "I'm not going on a cruise until I lose weight," she told me. (Some other life-pausing deprivations I've heard from others over the years: "I'll get divorced after I lose weight"; "I'll ask for a raise once I lose weight"; "I'll learn golf once I lose weight"; "I'll start my own business once I lose weight.") She didn't feel as if she could engage her whole self until she lost weight.

Were there ways to make her happy and kinder to her body, getting to a new mindset that chipped away at her mistaken beliefs—namely, that her weight was her worth; that weight defined her instead of being just one of many, many aspects of her; that weight and shape were central to who she was?

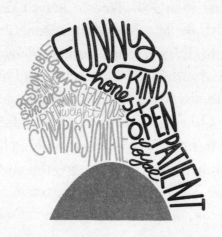

Was there a different way to look at herself, her body, and her life—or were the messages she'd incurred for so long about the overvaluing of weight and thinness, from people around her as well as society, simply too loud ever to overcome?

If she was going to have success on her weight-loss journey and, more importantly, develop a sense of herself independent of weight or shape, it was vital to help shore up how she felt about her body. Regardless of starting weight, those with a better body image when they begin a weight-loss journey are likelier to succeed than those with a poorer body image. In a word, they lose more weight. That might seem wildly counterintuitive. You might think that people who are critical of their bodies are more motivated and successful than those who aren't, but that's not the case.

It was important that she believe she was *not* her weight, so that she could separate it from who she was: a crucial mindset shift. One of the problems with negative body image is that it stops you from engaging in health-promoting activities. It can be so hard to step into a gym. If you have joint pain and the doctor tells you that swimming helps, what messages are you telling yourself about the imagined experience if you hate your body? As Ava progressed on her journey, she was going to eat better and move more and get generally healthier (lower her cholesterol, blood pressure, diabetes risk, etc.) and, yes, lose weight, this last factor the most tangible outcome, at least to others. It was important that she view weight as just one metric, not the only one, since there were other ways in which she would be getting healthier and doing positive, loving things for herself and her body.

There were multiple techniques I presented to Ava and some resonated with her. First, we started with an exercise where she tried to recall the compliments and other positive comments that people had made to her over the years, about her personality, her intelligence, her kind heart, her energy, and so much more. Any positive she could think of, not necessarily having to do with how her body looked. If done regularly, this exercise allows you to think differently about your body and yourself, and the words can become an affirmation, or mantra, in your mind. "One of the first things we do with our patients is just get them to find things about themselves that they love or enjoy," says Gary Bennett, professor of psychology and neuroscience at Duke University, whose research program designs, tests, and disseminates digital obesity treatments. "The biggest symptom of carrying excess weight is beating up on yourself. You have to treat yourself with a little bit of empathy." Granted, it's not easy. Many people need to write the affirmations down before they can get the interior conversation going. Many people need someone with whom to have the conversation.

We also tried a body-focused exercise. It wouldn't

be about whether she had lost the weight she wanted, or some of it, or none of it, but about somehow helping her get to a better place about her body and therefore a healthier, happier place, period. A technique I liked then (and now) focuses on and celebrates all the things your body *does*. The more you value your body's utility rather than its appearance, the less scorn you have for your physical self, the less fixated you are on weight as the primary/only measure. And, as studies show, when you have a better body image, you have greater overall well-being and are likelier to be physically active, which in turn makes your journey more likely a success.

This exercise was even harder than the first one. After all, if asked to describe our bodies, most of us immediately think about how we look, and usually focus on the part of our body we dislike most. Past experiences and comments may have caused you to have negative thoughts and emotions about your overall appearance or specific areas of your body. These thoughts and emotions may have been forming for so long that by now they seem automatic. This can undermine weight control—and, more important, your sense of self.

Imagine what it might be like if you woke up one morning and all of your unhelpful thoughts about your body were gone. You don't have to love it, but what if when you thought about your body, you stopped thinking about what was wrong with it? Instead, imagine how different it would feel if you thought about what your body *did*. What would that feel like? What would be different? What would you do differently? Ava needed to forget, at least for a moment, her displeasure with her body—the idea that a bigger body was "objectively" in her view an unattractive body—and instead focus on what it did for her.

How those thighs, which she hated, provided a strong base to carry her body as she climbed stairs and took care of patients all day as a nurse; those arms that were able to carry her kids, cook, and paint; that belly that protected her two children as they grew inside her.

The effort it takes to like your body is daunting. "Everything is going against you liking your body," says Dianne Neumark-Sztainer, Ph.D., professor at the University of Minnesota and an expert on body dissatisfaction, whose research focuses on the prevention and reduction of weight-related problems. "We get so many negative, judgmental cues throughout our lifetime, at key stages of our life." To offset this, you need to "accept that, yeah, there is always going to be someone faster, smarter, has better hair, whatever it may be, but you have lots of positive traits, too. Think about all the amazing things that you can do with your body."

Ava began to glimpse how she could show respect for her body, a belief in its value, just by taking care of it, by eating better, moving more, practicing mindfulness, stretching, getting regular sleep.

But it was hard. It didn't happen in one session.

There were setbacks. It wasn't the only change she was attempting to make.

Over time, Ava started to appreciate that her weight was not the whole of her. She still didn't like her arms but decided that, if she was going to compare herself to others, instead of looking at people's arms, she would look at their calves, because she liked the way her own calves looked. More importantly, she didn't have to see herself in constant relation to everyone else. She came to see that thin was not everything. "Healthy is the new skinny," as Oprah says.

In time—and it took time—her body image was less contingent on being a certain size or shape. Her body had value. She knew that she herself had fundamental value, independent of her weight or shape. There were ripple effects: How she felt about herself improved the way she ate, how she dressed, how she walked into a room. Though she wasn't the dress size she had initially said she "needed" to be to feel happy, though she hadn't lost the weight she had targeted before she could book a cruise, she decided to live her life now. She started wearing more oranges and pinks.

Stigma and Negative Body Image

When you live in a society that sends the message that your weight equals your worth, how do you uncouple what you weigh or how you think your body compares to others with your sense of self—who you are?

It can be done in ways that you have already seen, like practicing self-compassion (chapter 1), reality-checking unhelpful thinking styles (chapter 2), and leveraging your strengths (chapter 4).

It can also be done by changing the way you think about your own body.

Body image is just what it sounds like: how you perceive your body and your personal relationship with it, formed through all the beliefs, thoughts, feelings, and actions pertaining to your physical appearance. How you value it. Because you're with your body all the time, it's hard to feel good about yourself if you feel bad about your body.

People who have overweight or obesity are more likely to have a negative body image. Of course, there's no preset body image associated with a particular weight or body type: People who look the same shape and size to others can have quite different body images. Living in a larger body and body image are not in some exact inverse proportion, where the more you weigh, the less positive your body image. There are people who weigh three hundred pounds who have a positive body image, and those who weigh a hundred twenty pounds who have a negative one.

A lot of the variation in body image is based on cultural norms. For example, men have less negative body image than women, and Black women have less body image dissatisfaction than White women. Among various ethnic groups, greater levels of acculturation are associated with greater levels of body dissatisfaction.

The goal of this book and so much of my clinical work, which has often focused on weight- and shape-based stigma, is to help people gain awareness of the unhelpful body assumptions and errors they make. Once they learn to identify these negative thoughts when they occur, they can take steps to correct them.

It's your body image, but of course the influences on it are hardly yours alone. The three most significant factors that contribute to your body image are

- *Personal history*: what your parents, siblings, peers, etc., said to you when you were growing up, both positive and negative; teasing; incidents around puberty and dating; what people are saying now;
- *Culture*: the magazines you read, the social media you follow, the prejudices, biases, and discriminations that exist and are related to weight; "standards" about what is attractive and ideal;
- *Self-talk*: how you talk to yourself influences how you think and feel about yourself; comparing yourself to others.

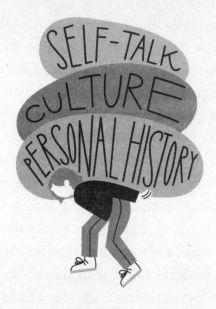

The influences on body image, as you can see, are far-flung and, way too often, potentially toxic. Those who live in a body that is larger than society deems "ideal" can internalize over the years lots of the unhelpful and nasty comments, the disappointed and disapproving looks. The erroneous assumptions that embed themselves in the mind—e.g., *my weight defines me*—are not easily erased. In her song, "You Say," Lauren Daigle powerfully and painfully captures how internalizing negative messages—about anything—becomes a constant, exhausting struggle for self-worth. "I keep fighting voices in my mind that say I'm not enough, Every single lie that tells me I will never measure up."

By the time I'd worked in the field of weight management for even just a few years, I had seen far too many examples of the awful piling on: not just the horrible stigmatization of my patients by their own circle and the larger world, but the scorn these individuals had for their own bodies, the way their body image defined their self-image. The internalizing of weight stigma becomes a lot about who you think you are as a person. It's not just that you think your body is too big, too this or too that, and you're certain that everyone thinks that, too; it's that you think everyone thinks you're lazy and weak and *that's* why your body looks like it does, so you think you're lazy and weak, too. It's about not only your weight and shape but also your character. It's your fault. You're a bad person. You have no worth outside of your weight and shape. It's a narrow view with wide-reaching consequences.

Of course, the revelation that negative body image could so often lead to negative self-image was dismaying to me. As a young clinician, I could see—as could many others working in the field—that this perception would be a significant barrier to self-compassion or an inspiring wellness journey. It was an eye-opener for me that a preoccupation with weight and shape fueled so many unhealthy habits. It was not a mindset conducive to happiness and health, never mind weight loss.

It's important to acknowledge just how heart-wrenching the experience of weight stigma can be, how hard it can be for people who weigh more than society deems "normal" to hold on to a positive self-image, one not wholly colored by weight, when the world seems to be telling them otherwise. The problem goes beyond the diminution of human value. It affects care. Something like this may have happened to you: You go to a doctor for a sinus infection or something else unrelated to body weight. The doctor addresses the "weight issue" while treating the sinus infection, perhaps even linking the two. "Your weight," you're told, "makes everything worse." That experience of receiving such a critique for something that may have nothing to do with weight makes patients less likely to seek health care. It increases negative self-talk, which in turn "can become a real threat to engagement, making people just turn away from care," says Duke's Bennett.

Far too many healthcare providers hold the misguided belief that their patients who have overweight or obesity did it to themselves, that they're lazy. One of my first studies on this topic found that over fifty percent of primary care physicians described patients who lived with obesity as "awkward," "unattractive," "ugly," and "non-compliant." Much more recently (in 2021), WW did a qualitative study, led by Dr. Lisa Bailey-Davis at Geisinger Health System, about physician practices in providing or referring for the treatment of obesity. We found that the main barrier for the doctors was the perception that their patients weren't "motivated." It's an unfortunate cycle that has consequences all around. Stigma can prevent people from doing the behaviors they need to do to "help" their health. And they suffer: According to a study led by Rebecca Puhl, Ph.D., professor at the University of Connecticut and the deputy director of its Rudd Center for Food Policy and Obesity, young adults who experienced weight stigma pre-pandemic had higher levels of depressive symptoms and stress, and were likelier to use eating as a coping strategy and to binge-eat during COVID-19 versus those who hadn't experienced weight stigma.

There's an assumption by far too many (often subconsciously) that those who have overweight or obesity got that way by eating unhealthily. While eating and activity habits can significantly change body weight, genetics is responsible for 40–70 percent of the variation in body weight. Simply put, people who eat the same and exercise the same do not necessarily weigh the same. Weight is not a standardized indicator of any personal characteristic. Yet despite these well-established facts, the chorus is clear: *It's your fault. You could do something about it if you really wanted.* People with overweight or obesity are frequently described as lacking discipline, having no willpower, being gluttonous. How do they absorb this cacophony and still value their body? How do they untie body image from self-worth? That's a lot of mind trash to clean up.

I'm not suggesting that there is no connection between weight and increased risk of stroke, diabetes, or other health conditions, or that these should be ignored. But the way even trained health professionals think they should and can talk to those who struggle with weight—as if there's nothing wrong with the content or tone of their communication—is mind-boggling and distressing. I once gave a medical grand rounds lecture, titled "Recent Developments in Obesity Treatment," at a prominent university. As I often do in such talks, I included a few slides on steps that physicians can take to accommodate larger-size patients, like procuring larger exam gowns, scales that measure above three hundred pounds, larger blood-pressure cuffs, and armless chairs or ones that are wide enough for larger people to sit in comfortably. During the Q&A, one physician commented that he was concerned that such measures would make people with obesity feel "too comfortable," and it was our role as health care professionals to create some discomfort to motivate change.

There it was: the pervasive bias and stigma against larger body sizes and the belief that shame leads to behavior change, all in one comment. In his view, obesity was simply a problem of motivation; shame was an effective motivator; you could weigh whatever you wanted if you really tried. I responded with a polite debunking of his thinking and tried to provide a different point of view, but underneath I felt crushed by the brutal reality of his comments. I was more motivated than ever to hold these myths to the light and expose their consequences so that people could get the care they deserve, with dignity.

Doctors are not alone in stigmatizing higher weight and bigger bodies. In one of our recent studies, family members were the most frequent actors in weight-based stigma, with classmates next.

Weight discrimination remains accepted by many, while other types of discrimination are regularly called out or criminalized. People still tell "fat jokes"—though, granted, fewer today than twenty years ago, and it's hard to imagine a popular show like *Friends*, were it created today, would have the Monica Geller (Courteney Cox) backstory: a teen girl with severe obesity whose size was played for straight-up laughs. Perfectly qualified job candidates are still often deprived of professional opportunities because of their weight, though it has nothing to do with their ability to perform the tasks of the job. It's not right to stigmatize any segment of society, no matter their number, but it's incredible to consider that the group being stigmatized here accounts for *more than 70 percent of the adult American population.*

It requires no great leap to conclude that individuals internalize society's underlying message. "What we see from the mass media, from societal messages about weight from the diet industry and the fashion industry, is that this really does come down to personal effort," says Puhl. "However, we know from considerable science that this is just not the case: Body weight is a very complex issue that is caused by many different factors outside of your personal control. But we don't hear those messages very often. And as a result of this societal weight stigma, these kinds of stereotypes remain very prevalent." To take one influential example: Puhl points out that anti-bullying policies for schools admirably call out and codify other common areas of stigmatization that place youth at risk for bullying—race, gender, religion, disability, etc.—"but when it comes to weight, policy language is often absent. Many other forms of stigma have legitimate movements that have been very vocal, where policy now prohibits unfair treatment based on characteristics like gender or race. But it remains legal to discriminate on the basis of weight." A scan of anti-bullying policies at 9,000+ school districts across America reveals that weight doesn't even register among the top eighteen listed categories; "appearance" is tenth, but that can include a host of traits, such as hair, clothing, piercings, complexion, etc.

Besieged by the critical reactions from loved ones, health care providers, and the culture at large, it's no wonder that so many people with overweight make faulty assumptions about their appearance, leading to a negative body image. The four items below, adapted from *The Body Image Workbook* by Tom Cash, Ph.D., one of the pioneers in the field, represent the top false beliefs held by people with a negative body image:

1. Physically attractive people have it all.
2. The first thing that people will notice about me is what's wrong with my appearance.
3. If I could look just as I wish, my life would be much happier.
4. The only way I could ever like my looks would be to change them.

These echo the internal beliefs I hear expressed most frequently—but because I work with people who have overweight and obesity, their perceptions are weight-based:

1. Thin people have it all.
2. The first thing people notice about me is my weight.
3. If I lost weight, I would be happier.
4. The only way I (or anyone) can like my body is for me to lose weight.

The leap is painfully easy to make. As Puhl puts it, "internalizing stigma happens when people become aware of weight-based stereotypes around them, apply those beliefs to themselves, and engage in self-directed stigma or personal blame."

In Cash's workbook he also describes what he calls "ugly errors in your private body talk." He characterizes these errors into eight categories that are common for a variety of body image concerns. Based on my clinical experience, four of Cash's thinking styles are most prevalent among those with whom I've worked. Do any of these sound familiar?

1. **BEAUTY OR BEAST:** You view your appearance in terms of extremes—and usually extremes based on weight. Thoughts like *I can look good only after I lose fifty pounds* are typical. This is a variant of all-or-none thinking, discussed in chapter 2 but applied to your body.

2. **UNFAIR TO COMPARE:** You compare yourself to others but only on the aspect of your body that you like least. For example, if you're unhappy with the size of your arms, you'll compare yourself only to people who have arms that you consider to be more attractive.

3. **MAGNIFYING GLASS:** You focus on a feature of your appearance that you don't like and magnify its importance. You look in the mirror and the only thing you can see is the thing you dislike most, ignoring every other aspect of your body and what it does for you. This is similar to the negative filter discussed in chapter 2.

4. **BEAUTY BOUND:** You decree that you can't do certain things because of how you look or what you weigh. Examples include "I can't go to the beach / go on a cruise / wear bright colors until I lose weight."

At the end of this chapter there are techniques to identify and modify these types of thinking.

No evidence exists that body self-hate "works" to get to you to a better place. *The more I hate my body, the better I'll do* is untrue. It's hard to find lasting success on a weight-loss journey if you have a negative body image. We know from our recent studies that internalized weight bias is associated with *less* weight loss, eating self-efficacy, self-monitoring, body image, and quality of life; and *more* weight gain, weight cycling, stress, and eating to cope.

A good deal of my work has been devoted to exposing the falsehood that hating your body would better fuel the journey, and promoting the fact that self-compassion and valuing your body tend to lead to improved results. WW is working with two prominent researchers in the field, Drs. Rebecca Puhl and Rebecca Pearl, to understand how weight stigma affects our members in the United States and globally and how we can help decrease its impact and internalization.

I'm aware, though, that addressing something as profound as weight stigma—how it makes you feel and what it makes you do—is a tall order to be resolved in a book chapter or two. To explore more resources on weight stigma, here are some important organizations:

- UConn Rudd Center for Food Policy and Obesity
- Obesity Action Coalition
- Association for Size Diversity and Health

I Want to Lose Weight . . . *and* I Value My Body

How can the seemingly contradictory ideas above both be true? The notion of weight loss seems to suggest you'd be better off if you were thinner. If that were so, then how can you value your body as it is, if the bottom line is that less weight is generally superior? Isn't that buying *precisely* into weight-based stigma?

A weight-loss journey is not exclusively or even largely about "looking better." It's about you wanting to do the best you can for your body, improving the way your body functions. Weight loss and changes in body image are frequent outcomes of taking better care of yourself and your body. There are important reasons, having nothing to do with looks, for why someone who has lost weight tends to feel better about their body. You move in space better. Perhaps you sit more comfortably in an airplane seat. You walk up steps without shortness of breath. You can stand for extended periods without pain. You're able to play tag with your kids or grandkids and catch up to them. You can ride on a rollercoaster. Your health improves.

To enable all these positive outcomes—through healthy eating, physical activity, better sleep—is an act of kindness to yourself, not criticism. It's an act of valuing, not devaluing. The physical changes— "improvements"—in your body that many experience with weight loss will make your body feel better. You have fundamental value, and therefore your body does, too.

Compared to other physical conditions, there's an element to weight loss and body image that's unique. Weight and bodies get "graded" differently, usually more harshly, than other aspects of an individual's physical, mental, emotional, intellectual, and moral being. People with diabetes don't typically say, "I hate my pancreas." People with asthma don't hate their lungs or see themselves as unworthy of love. The presence of more weight or less weight in a given person is visible to the outside world; your pancreas and lungs are not. When you lose weight, your body looks different, in ways that are generally more socially acceptable. As I wrote above, weight loss almost always improves one's body image. We know this from studies, including my own; I know this from my own clinical experience. Yet so much more than weight loss can impact your overall body image.

When we ask people around the globe about their

wellness goals, yes: The vast majority include weight loss in their answer—not surprising, given the high global prevalence of overweight and obesity. For them, weight loss is a way to improve their wellness, but it's not the only way. That's why we don't tell people how much weight to lose. We don't tell them to hit a certain BMI. You set your goal weight. You can set a goal weight that's five pounds away, then add to it later. Or not. We won't tell you how much to weigh because our role is to help you reach your individual wellness goal, whatever it is. Valuing your body does not preclude you wanting to improve some "usable" aspect of it—your mobility, your flexibility, your stamina. If weight loss is the goal, then we help you make the behavior changes necessary to achieve that. If your goal is to eat more fruits and vegetables, then we help you understand the "how" (see chapter 3) of making that happen. If you're looking to get a smaller belly for your thirtieth high school reunion, you can succeed at getting there. Cosmetic changes can make people happy. I am not diminishing anyone's enthusiasm to "look good" or "look better." Patients and members come in all the time saying things like, "My belly is too big" or "I want to be able to fit into the jeans I bought pre-pregnancy" or "I want to zip boots over my calves" or a hundred other discrete physical/cosmetic goals. Early in my career, I was judgmental about such motivations, thinking they wouldn't lead to lasting change. The more experience and interactions I had as a clinician and as a human being, though, the more I learned that people's reasons are their reasons. Cosmetic changes are real and important for some. If that were a patient's motivation, then I needed to jump on board and help her/him get where she/he wanted to go. I believed—and still do—that if the change being sought is motivated mostly by the desire to look better, in a way more consistent with many societal standards, then the change is not likely to last. If, on the other hand, the change is motivated mostly by the person's desire to treat their body kindly or to feel better in their own skin, then the chance for lasting success is greater.

The reason to make behavior change is to live a happier, healthier life; that entails eating differently, moving differently, and thinking differently; that entails being kind to your body and yourself. To the extent that a successful journey *also* results in weight loss? Great, if it makes you happy, and that was one of your goals.

This turns the dilemma inside out: Your weight and wellness journey is about what is good for you and your body, *not* about your body being deficient and needing fixing. The weight-loss outcome, in and of itself, will not be enough. If the driving force behind the journey is to treat your body well and make it and you feel good, that's likely to last.

You've surely heard the expression "treat your body

like a temple." It's worthy of respect, even reverence. That applies to any weight and size.

Benefits of a More Positive Body Image

Developing a positive body image provides significant benefits:

- It helps you appreciate your body and feel good about the changes you're making.
- It gives you a tool that isn't food to help manage/minimize the negative thoughts related to your body (*my legs are too big, my arms are flabby,* etc.) that can disrupt healthy eating and activity habits.
- Those with a positive body image "binge-eat" and overeat less frequently than those with a negative body image.
- A more positive body image is linked to more successful long-term weight-loss outcomes.
- An improved body image is associated with better quality of life.

Though the following techniques have been shown to work, your body image won't change in a day or a week. It may be difficult to know which one is for you. You may feel a technique is not working because you simply can't *not* think about your body.

I understand. It's completely normal. How we think about our bodies is ingrained; after all, we have a life-long history with them. It takes time and practice to shift mindset. It's unlikely that you're just going to "flip a switch" and feel great about your body over-night. Once you do get going with a technique, be patient and realistic about how long it will take to change. Progress is more important than perfection. Even making the decision to *try* to think differently about your body is a move in the right direction. If you feel frustrated with yourself, go back to the self-compassion techniques in chapter 1.

You may even lose weight yet feel as if you don't see real improvement in your body image. This, too, is normal. It's going to take time.

As long as you're doing something for yourself, not against yourself; doing something positive, not puni-tive; starting from a position of strength, not weak-ness, then you're on the right path to a better body image and a better journey.

My Shift: Kaitlyn

My body is not the enemy. Before I had my daughter I would critique myself, pick myself apart. And don't get me wrong: I still have my insecurities. I still can think, *Oh, I wish my belly didn't look that way* or, *Oh, I need to lose another five pounds*, or, *I need to do this or do that*. But after having my daughter and seeing the way my body grew another human and cared for her and then I breastfed for seven months, how in the world can I be mad at my body now? How in the world can my body be the enemy after seeing this crazy, beautiful thing it's done? That clicked for me. Rather than kicking myself and abusing myself like—I don't want to say awful language . . . you wouldn't talk to your best friend that way, yet you're talking to yourself like that. *Look at the way you look today*. Rather than doing that, it clicked. *Okay, what can you do to really care for yourself today?* Like eating healthy foods or exercising that makes me feel good. That's what I'm going to choose today rather than *I'm going to exercise because I really want to get to one-sixty*. That mindset shift was big.

Suddenly, here you are with a newborn and you're on their time. That's when it hit me, Okay, this is what I'm going to do to love on myself and take care of my body. And I just didn't look back.

SKILL BUILDING FOR VALUING YOUR BODY: THE TECHNIQUES

What You Do for Me

If asked to describe our bodies, many of us would immediately think about how we look. And because most cultures have unrealistic ideals for how we "should" look, focusing on our body's appearance can contribute to an unhelpful body image. Use this technique to begin to shift the narrative away from how your body looks towards what it does. It's okay and completely normal for it to take time for this activity to come naturally. Be patient with yourself and remember that you deserve compassion. The more regularly you practice the technique, the more likely your thoughts will shift.

1. **TAKE A MOMENT TO VISUALIZE A PART OF YOUR BODY THAT YOU WISH WAS DIFFERENT.** If you typically think, *My arms are so big*, take a moment to picture your arms. It doesn't have to be your least favorite body part—choose one that you feel comfortable thinking about.

2. **NEXT, THINK ABOUT HOW YOU USE THIS PART OF YOUR BODY AND WHAT IMPORTANT ROLE IT PLAYS.** Put aside notions of how it looks or what you don't like about it.

What can you accomplish with it that matters to you? Your arms may help you carry heavy things, throw a ball, or hug your loved ones. Your legs may help you walk through a museum or supermarket or mall, or to explore nature.

3. **CREATE AN AFFIRMATION TO RECOGNIZE HOW THAT BODY PART HELPS YOU AND WHAT IT CAN ACCOMPLISH.** My arms help me because they give me the opportunity to carry groceries, hug my partner, or lift my child.

   My legs help me explore museums and nature, which feeds my love of learning.

4. **ONCE YOU HAVE YOUR AFFIRMATION, SAY IT TO YOURSELF IN YOUR MIND ONCE A DAY.**

Reality Check

Identifying and countering the unhelpful thoughts related to your body are key to your success. If this technique feels familiar, that's because you've seen it in chapter 2. Just like Reality Checks can help you shift unhelpful thoughts about your journey, they can also be used to shift unhelpful thoughts related to your body.

1. **I.D. AN UNHELPFUL THOUGHT.** Ask yourself, *What are my thoughts about my body right now? What is the*

story I'm telling myself about my body? An example: Your friend invites you to the beach. You think, *There's no way I can have fun at the beach and be seen in a bathing suit right now!*

2. **DO A REALITY CHECK.** You can do this in two different ways. The first is to pretend you're a lawyer. Ask yourself, *Are there facts to back up my thought? What's the evidence to support it? What facts demonstrate that this thought is not true?* For example, *Is it true that I really can't have fun at the beach? Is it impossible for me to be seen in a bathing suit?* Or ask yourself, *If a friend shared this thought, what would I say to her? How would I help her feel comfortable going to the beach?*

3. **RESPOND TO YOUR REALITY CHECK WITH A NEW HELPFUL THOUGHT.** Based on the answers to your reality check, is there another, more helpful way to think about the situation? For example, *How I think about my body doesn't need to dictate whether I have fun at the beach. I can go to the beach and do things I love with my friends.*

In the following chart, you'll find examples based on Tom Cash's thought distortions that lead to negative body image. These are the unhelpful thoughts that I hear most frequently. The examples may help you to identify your own thoughts, perform reality checks, and develop alternative, helpful thoughts.

THINK AGAIN		
Beauty or Beast: You regard your appearance in terms of extremes. You may not be happy with yourself if you are somewhere between these two extremes.	Unhelpful thought	"I will look good only when I reach my goal weight."
	Reality check	"Is reaching a certain weight the only measure of success? Isn't it possible to look good right now? Weight loss is a continual journey, so why would I expect a change only when I reach some distant goal?"
	Helpful thought	"I am making great progress. Just because I haven't reached the weight I want doesn't mean my body isn't starting to change. My weight is not the only thing that defines my body. It does so many great things for me."
Unfair to Compare: You compare yourself to people around you, usually picking things you like least about yourself to serve as the standard of comparison.	Unhelpful thought	"That woman has such small thighs. My thighs are so big, I wish they looked like hers."
	Reality check	"Does the fact that her thighs look small mean mine must be big? How does she set the standard for how I should look? Does this woman's appearance relate to my own?"
	Helpful thought	"The fact that I like how that woman's thighs look does not mean mine look big. Everybody has different attributes. Some bigger, some smaller, some the same."

The Magnifying Glass: You focus on a feature of your appearance that you don't like and "magnify" its importance.	Unhelpful thought	"I know I've lost weight but my belly is still too big and I don't look good."
	Reality check	"Am I really going to let such a small aspect of my appearance ruin how great I feel in this outfit today?"
	Helpful thought	"My belly may not be perfect but it's not going to ruin my day. I am treating my body well and I look and feel good."
Beauty Bound: You cannot do certain things because of your looks.	Unhelpful thought	"I can't buy stylish clothes until I lose twenty pounds."
	Reality check	"Why can't I? Is there a rule somewhere that says people who are heavier than they'd like can't wear stylish clothes? Should others decide what I wear?
	Helpful thought	"Just because I'm not at a certain weight doesn't mean I can't be stylish. I'm not going to wait to be stylish. I deserve to wear things I like."

——————— ADDITIONAL RESOURCES ———————

- *The Body Image Workbook, Second Edition,* by Thomas Cash
- *Living with Your Body & Other Things You Hate: How to Let Go of Your Struggle with Body Image Using Acceptance & Commitment Therapy* by Emily Sandoz
- Podcast: What is Weight Stigma? with Dr. Rebecca Puhl on Factually! With Adam Conover

What's Next

Losing weight alone is unlikely to change how you feel fundamentally about your body. Treating your body with dignity rather than disdain will serve you and your body well over the long haul. Another kindness that will serve you well is getting the support you deserve from others (for those who want and need it).

The next chapter shows you why and how to do that.

I DESERVE TO ~~GO IT ALONE~~ GET THE SUPPORT I NEED

Finding Your People

It's a family dinner, you're trying to eat healthier (more greens, baked chicken instead of fried), and several of the people around the table are rolling their eyes at your efforts. None of them have tried to lose weight before. You eat a dinner roll you didn't want, just to deflect the attention.

Saturday night out with friends, you're being more intentional about what you order, but they don't seem to be, and you're afraid they'll see you as a wet blanket. You buy an extra round of drinks to show your spirit, downing yours quickly.

At a farewell party for a coworker, the host wraps up an extra piece of homemade cake for you (you had a slice during the toasts); you politely decline, but she insists. You don't want to insult her. You take the slice home.

The time chunks you set aside for being active bump up against of-the-moment demands of others in your life—spouse/partner, children, friends, colleagues. You miss all but one of the slots you'd set aside to work out during the week.

Examples like these don't happen on just one day or one night or one meal or one week. They happen all the time. After all, the people in your life need to be considered, accommodated. They care about you and want what's best for you (most of them, anyway)—but often they don't know how to help. And as much as you may benefit from having them in your corner, you may also struggle to communicate what kind of social support would work best, for both your weight-management journey and the relationship you share.

What do I mean by "social support"? At its most basic, it's the network of people who provide you with acknowledgment, encouragement, specific information, and resources to help you succeed.

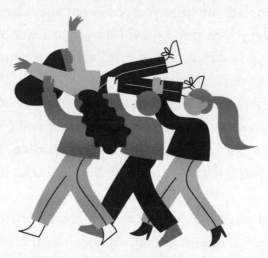

It can mean companionship or a check-in or words that emotionally and psychologically nurture. A core element to recruiting social support is simply telling people what you need from them and also "correcting" what they're doing when it's not working. How do you cope with people in your social circle who are not being supportive? If, say, your partner doesn't know how to help you, can you just give up on getting support from them and ignore everything that's unhelpful, and simply decide not to ask them for their help? You could, but their actions—or lack of action—still influence you.

Others can help or hurt your progress. That sentence can excite and encourage you, or it can terrify and deflate you. Just how, or how much, the actions and words of others affect you depends a lot on your mindset. That's not to suggest that you're at the mercy of others. In fact, you can influence how they support you. That may seem a bit daunting, at first. But it's something you can learn and master, and its benefits transcend lasting weight loss.

It's one thing to shift your own routines and mindset, but what is it like when other people are also involved in the shift? Seeking support is not just about your shift but theirs, too. You want the most effective support, of course, but in the often delicate process of sharing what you seek, you also want the other person to feel valued, and not have them or you feel judged.

This chapter will give you the overview and skills to shift your mindset so that you can get the support you need and deserve rather than be at the whims of others.

While some people on a weight-loss journey don't see the need for social support, it provides meaningful psychological health benefits. "Early on, we didn't quite realize how important social support is for weight-loss success," says Amy Gorin, Ph.D., professor at the University of Connecticut and a leading researcher in the social influences on weight, eating, and physical activity, "so people would come in to lose weight and we looked at them very much as an individual, talked to them about what they could do individually to change their diet and exercise and mostly ignored the larger context in which people live, work, and socialize. For the longest time we mentioned to people that it was helpful to get friends and family members on board with their weight-loss goals, but we only scratched this concept at the surface. We now understand that people are heavily influenced by those around them, especially when it comes to weight and eating and exercise behaviors. And that it's critical to leverage the support of people around you when you're trying to make health behavior change. Otherwise, you're learning new weight-management skills or trying to establish new behavioral habits in a vacuum, and as soon as you go back to your existing social environments, you're bound to regain or struggle."

(This doesn't mean you *must* have social support to succeed; I'll discuss "going solo" later in the chapter.)

Indeed, not only do the words, actions, and mere presence of others affect you; yours affect them. What is known in weight-loss circles as "the ripple effect" refers to how, when one spouse/partner follows a structured weight-management program, the other one tends to lose weight, too. This was shown in a 2018 study of WW members, as well as in several other studies.

Why and Who

Science has shown that when you have people in your corner, it helps in weight- and wellness-specific ways. Individuals with social support are

- more likely to engage in behaviors of healthy eating and physical activity;
- less likely to regain weight or turn back to behaviors of unhealthy eating or unhealthy physical activity;
- more likely to lose weight—those who receive the most social support from friends and family

lose more weight at six months versus those who get little or no support.

The science on the impact of social support is so powerful, *community* is built into the WW experience. WW's members-only social platform, Connect, is an example of people supporting people. Users cheer each other on when they reach milestones on the scale or beyond, or share comfort over a challenging experience, which may lead to helpful new information and perspective. ("I find tracking tedious" . . . "Did you ever put a stopwatch on it? It only takes 4.3 minutes a day" . . . "Try tracking just a little; that worked for me.") The conversations on Connect can get profound. Members have been helped through tragedies—the loss of parents, spouses, even children—by their Connect friends.

How do you know what kind and level of support work best for you?

Gorin suggests asking yourself, "What type of support or encouragement do I tend to respond well to in other areas of my life, like work or school?" Then "apply that to the weight management process."

In finding support, there's always a what and a who. First, define what would be supportive for you. What is it you want? To take Gorin's example, think about areas/relationships in your life where you feel good and supported and happy. Perhaps it looks and feels something like these scenarios:

- someone notices you're stressed and asks what they can do to help;
- a coworker pitches in because you're up against a deadline;
- a family member offers to take the kids overnight just to give you a break;
- a colleague reaches out after a tough meeting just to see how you're doing;
- you say to your spouse/partner, "This is not a good time to discuss this"—and they don't.

Then you need to define who can and will help you: family members, friends, those on a similar journey? If those people care about you but aren't helping in this way, how can you help them help you? You'll need to tell them exactly what you need—and don't need—them to do for you.

If you don't have an existing circle, where might you find like-minded, supportive, nonjudgmental people to help?

There are two pools of possible support: people you know and people you don't yet know who might be particularly helpful. Social support need not suggest a vast, many-tentacled network. It's about having someone in your life who understands what you're aiming to do and can provide you with help in achieving your goals. It's a simple, powerful experience: You need a person (or people) in your corner to support you, and you need to "manage" the relationship so that they in fact help and don't unintentionally harm your progress.

My Shift: Ginger

I have an Instagram account where I post all my journeys about food and fitness. I follow people in other countries and they follow me.

Through that I've met people who have struggled with their weight for years, who have children who struggle with their weight, or just overall need the accountability because it's easier when you do it with a group. It branched out and I met more people and made new connections, and honestly it's been awesome. I appreciate that it's people I've never met, complete strangers, who will clap for me just like anyone else.

What I learned from community is that it wasn't just a number on a scale. It was more than the weight loss. I've befriended people who like the same books, or the same shoe brands, or who have done similar workout programs. That's helped it to branch out into more of a community because it's not just, *Oh, you have 20 pounds to lose? I have 20 pounds to lose!* It's what else are we also doing and learning about each other along the way?

My friend Julie and I were sending each other pictures of our food. It was fun. There was no pressure behind it from either of us. When I hit my goal, she was as excited for me as I was, and it wasn't like there was any jealousy or fomo.

Without the support, I'm not sure I would have had the same drive or motivation. There are times I'm stuck on a plateau or feel like I'll never get past a certain point. And there's always someone, whether it's my mom, or someone else in my family, or friends outside of that from work or school who will say, "You can do this, you will achieve it." Without that I feel like there would have been a lot more times of me quitting. I might not have hit PLAY on that workout.

Potential Barriers

Before you learn the techniques that make it easier to enlist support and to have it be effective: Do you think you need support in the first place? Do you think it will make things easier? Do you think you deserve it?

So many individuals on a weight-management journey have a mindset that enforces the idea that they have no right to receive support. Or they get support and know they deserve it but struggle dealing with well-meaning people who are not in fact helping (e.g., the otherwise dear aunt who thinks that forcing food on you is loving and harmless, while you can't bring yourself to tell her how this messes with your progress). Or some people believe that they don't deserve better support from a *particular* individual in their life (e.g., they may get support from their friends, say, but not so much from their partner, and have resolved that it's not right to ask for more). Their mindset is telling them—with faulty evidence, and often little self-compassion—that it ultimately falls 100 percent on them to "fix" themselves.

> *I don't deserve more help than what people are willing to give.*
>
> *It's selfish to ask for help.*
>
> *My progress doesn't matter to others.*
>
> *No one will ever understand this journey I'm on.*
>
> *People who haven't been in my shoes can't help.*
>
> *I should be able to do it on my own.*
>
> *I don't ask my coworkers to do my job for me, so why ask others to help with this?*
>
> *My weight, my responsibility.*
>
> *I should have the willpower.*

I should be able to look a cake eye to eye and win that fight.

Somehow a solo victory, certain people believe, counts more than a supported one. Asking for help is a sign of weakness. They're embarrassed to ask for help, even in a small way. Instead, they isolate, resolving to grit and grind through it on their own.

Cheryl felt she had to brute-strength her way through weight loss. "This is not my husband's problem," she told me. "It's not my children's problem."

"Do you help them with anything?" I asked.

She looked at me as if I had three heads. "Of course."

"Tell me how. Tell me what you do for them."

After she had ticked off about a dozen items, I stopped her. "Cheryl, it seems like what you said to me a couple minutes ago, about losing weight, is really important to you," I said.

"It is."

"Why is it important to you?"

"I want to be around for my kids. For when they get married. I want to meet my grandchildren. I want to be a good role model for my kids."

"Okay. And it sounds like losing weight is more difficult when your husband and your kids do things that don't really support the effort, and may even get in the way."

"Yes."

"Would you say you're worth asking help for?"

She paused before nodding.

Like Cheryl, many of those who are on a weight-loss journey will refrain from seeking support. They're often beset by thoughts or beliefs that hold them back from getting—or even seeking—advice. Do any of these thoughts sound familiar?

I'm scared of failing in front of an audience.

I don't want the people in my life policing my choices.

My weight loss is too personal to share.

Let's just take the last one. It's a totally normal sentiment, yet seeking support doesn't have to mean divulging every personal detail of your journey. Instead of telling your friend that you're trying to lose thirty pounds, you could say, "I set a goal of walking on the town track for thirty minutes every other day. Can I put you on my list of walking buddies?" How much you share is up to you.

The Power of Specificity

The above beliefs can entrench a mindset that keeps you from seeking support and gaining its many benefits. Once you get past the internal angst over *Should I or shouldn't I ask for help?*, some of the basics to keep in mind:

Get specific. "I'd like you to be supportive." That sounds nice, but what does it really mean? The supporter has a lot of work to figure out what to do. Should they ask, "How much weight did you lose this week?" or "Should you be having cake on your 'diet'? Is that on your plan?" Should the questions be asked daily or weekly? If you tell your supporter, "Tell me when you see me with something I shouldn't eat," it's undefined about what should or shouldn't be eaten, and bound to cause trouble for both parties because it's so rich with implied judgment.

Your people want to help you, but they may just be guessing. Once you figure out what you need, fill them in. You're probably not looking for an evaluation of your behavior or a commentary on your journey, but for supportive behavior that responds to targeted questions or reminders that help you make the change you want. Something like, "If you could do the dishes this evening so I can take a walk, that would be great" or "If you put the cookies in the cabinet rather than on the counter, that would be amazingly helpful."

Lacking specifics and parameters, the supporter is likely to miss the mark. Being specific also helps shape your feedback on specific behaviors such as "I've noticed the cookies on the counter" rather than general characterizations such as "You haven't been support-ive!" or "You're a terrible spouse!"

I can't emphasize it enough: the more specific, the better.

Engage the right people. A rule of thumb for get-ting useful support: The closer the person is to you—someone you see or communicate with every day, or nearly that—the more you benefit from having "the discussion." If somebody is making it harder for you to succeed at your goal and the frequency of the exposure and/or importance of the relationship is great, you need to talk. On the other hand, if it's Aunt Millie, whom you see only at Thanksgiving, when she invariably tries to shove food down your throat, a conversation about how she can help you may be more trouble than it's worth.

You may also wish to choose as a supporter some-one on a similar path. It seems reasonable that your journey would be more successful if you partnered with a friend, spouse, or other companion also trying to lose weight, both of you motivating and encourag-ing each other to achieve a goal you both know all too well. Very often it works. Being on the same path fa-cilitates shared experiences and a deeper appreciation of the ups and downs of the process. And people on similar journeys can provide a much-needed reality check when thoughts turn to the unrealistic and the self-lacerating. "Peer accountability" is a major draw for many WW members because it enables them to find meaningful support from people outside their current circle.

Beware, though: What helps in your journey might not help in your supporter's. When you feel great, that person might be having a particularly rough time, or vice versa. That divergence can be useful for perspective and balance; however, especially if you share a household with your journey mate, be attentive, because if one of you goes off track, the other might follow.

You're worth helping, simple as that. So ask yourself: Are you likelier to succeed with the help of others? If you, like so many others, say yes, then rally the troops on your behalf!

Dealing with Saboteurs

Some people in your life—either ones you choose for support or not—may be witting, or more likely unwitting, saboteurs. They behave in a way that's counterproductive. Even some of the most well-meaning people can hurt your progress, derailing your weight-related efforts. Most of the time they don't know they're doing harm and, in fact, may think they're helping. I can't tell you how many people have shared with me a version of, "I'm going to ask my husband/wife/partner to help me with keeping track of what I ate"; when I see them next, they tell me, "The first time he/she 'helped' me, they asked if I measured my portions. It drove me up a wall!"

Because so many people mean to do well but lack knowledge about how, it's critical for *you* to decide what, specifically, is helpful to you (as stated earlier); then ask for that; then follow up (as described in one of the techniques at the end of this chapter). Be patient. It may take several requests and follow-ups to help those around you master the skills to help you effectively.

What about potential supporters who, despite your having made multiple requests and having provided feedback, persist in doing things that aren't helpful? This requires a more complex discussion. It's best to start with facts. "I've noticed that I've asked you a few times to avoid making comments about my weight or what I eat, but it still seems to be happening." (It may help here to cite one or two specific instances.) "What's getting in the way? Can you help me understand that?" These can be difficult conversations, but they're necessary: There's usually something underlying the behavior. Perhaps your "supporter" finds your weight-loss journey unsettling. It could be that they, too, want to engage in healthier behaviors but aren't in the right place to do so at the moment, making the juxtaposition between the two of you stark and uncomfortable. Maybe your weight and changed behavior have altered some fundamentals in your relationship (e.g., sexual intimacy, how food in general or certain foods in particular are no longer a means for socializing together). A change in weight, especially when it's considerable, could threaten your romantic partner, who hears positive, sometimes flirtatious comments directed at you from others as a threat.

It's not your job to figure out the reason. Your relationship is best served by creating a noncritical environment where frank, productive discussions can occur.

Who Are Your People?

Before identifying the challenges you need support for, you want to identify who "your people" are. What qualities are particularly high on your list? For example, you may feel you need someone who

- really listens to you;
- is optimistic but practical;
- empathizes even when they can't relate;
- has tackled a meaningful project;
- "gets" you whenever the two of you talk;
- makes you look forward to seeing/talking to them;

- makes you feel better after the two of you have talked;
- is available at odd hours;
- is not judgy.

This is a sample list. What are your must-haves in a supporter? Make a list of the top qualities you desire, then think of the people you're considering reaching out to. See how many checks they get on your wish list.

This quiz—in *The LEARN Program for Weight Management*, by my colleague Kelly Brownell, Ph.D., Duke University professor and a pioneer in the field of obesity and food policy—may also help you to recognize better if the person you're considering as your social support is right for you.

1. It is easy to talk to my partner about weight.
   True—5   False—1

2. My partner has always been thin and does not understand my weight problem.
   True—1   False—3

3. My partner offers me food when he or she knows I am trying to lose weight.
   True—1   False—5

4. My partner never says critical things about my weight.
   True—3   False—1

5. My partner is always there when I need a friend.
   True—4   False—1

6. When I lose weight and look better, my partner will be jealous.
   True—1   False—3

7. My partner will be genuinely interested in helping me with my weight.
   True—6   False—1

8. I could talk to my partner even if I was doing poorly.
   True—5   False—1

If you scored between 30 and 34, you may have found the perfect partner. A score in this range indicates that you and this person are comfortable with one another and can work together.

If you scored between 25 and 29, your friend is potentially a good partner, but there are areas of concern. Try asking the partner to take the quiz and predict how you answered the questions. This may help you make a decision.

If you scored between 17 and 24, there are areas of potential conflict, and a partnership with this person could encounter stormy going. Think of another partner.

If you scored between 8 and 16, definitely look to someone else as a partner. A partnership in this case would be a high-risk undertaking.

What If You Prefer Going Solo?

Maybe you're an introvert. Or just not a joiner. What if you have social support available to you but would rather go it alone? Is it possible to succeed solo on a weight-management journey?

Of course. No one size fits all. Although self-compassion is close to a necessity for a successful journey, there are those who "prefer to be held accountable by people in their lives when they go off their plan, and that works for them," says Gorin. "For other people, that undermines their effort." Those who go solo can reach their wellness goals. While some people thrive with a "support buddy," others find it more trouble than it's worth. Those going solo may find abundant benefit and inspiration in the writings, videos, podcasts, and other resources of people who've had similar life experiences and faced similar challenges. You don't have to interact with people directly to feel a kinship with their experience, which helps normalize your own and inspires you to keep going. Maybe it helps to surf message boards and online forums, feeling no pressure to share (at least until you're ready). Just seeing other people's posts can be helpful and affirming. One of the benefits of being part of a bigger group is that keeping your thoughts, concerns, and fears completely to yourself can often undermine success, while exposure, even anonymous, to a larger community and its pool of shared experience may prove comforting, validating, and motivating.

If you live with one or more persons, it can be more difficult to succeed without engaging them in some fashion. It's not about willpower. It's about your environment, and manipulating it so you're set up for success. If you live alone, you may have the "advantage" of not having somebody next to you eating ice cream or keeping their snack foods in open sight in the kitchen. If you live with someone, it's almost a non-negotiable that you'll need to involve them in things they can do or stop doing to make it easier for you to succeed.

Speak for Yourself: A Few Words About "No" and Boundary Setting

---

We're often asked to do things that conflict with our needs and goals: to go to an event we don't want to or don't have time for; to help with something we don't have the energy, enthusiasm, or skill to help with; to eat something we truly don't want when offered. Even when we're pretty sure it's best to say no, we often say yes anyway, or avoid responding altogether. We worry that saying no is impolite, unkind, selfish, that it will have a negative impact on the relationship. We're conditioned through cultural norms and family values to put others first; for the most part, human beings tend to try to avoid having negative feelings or being perceived negatively by others. Such avoidance often leads to decisions that are inconsistent with our intention.

Saying no is *not* inherently impolite, unkind, or selfish. What's more, it can be done effectively, in a way that respects and even benefits the relationship. When it comes to your own body and health, setting boundaries means prioritizing what you want over what others want for themselves or for you (though, in the end, the outcome may be what others want, too). This internal struggle is often felt particularly sharply during holidays and major social events, when we're often "keeping up" with friends and family traditions, and meeting the expectations of others.

The truth is, setting boundaries can help your relationships because it helps you. A "yes" to an event where you feel distracted, stressed, and resentful does you no good, and the person to whom you felt obligated will likely feel your less-than-all-in presence. You're upset. Now they're upset. It's not the outcome either of you had hoped for.

Still, it's hard to say no, especially to someone close. When done in a kind, thoughtful way, though, you're actually *growing* the relationship. In a sense, you're building or expanding your social support. Often, people consider their social support to mean simply this: *Do I have a good family? Do I have some-*

one in my corner? Are people in my circle doing things that help me or hurt me? In setting boundaries, such as saying no to an event, you're not merely putting your needs first and identifying what you yourself are gaining (e.g., *I'll have more time to take care of myself if I say no to this get-together*), but improving relationships. In doing that, you're taking charge of an even more robust network.

Nor must you view boundary setting as a yes-no switch. For example, if you find the holidays stressful because you do *all* the cooking for the family meals, set a boundary that you will make only three dishes and enlist help with the rest. Or challenge yourself (to give a few examples) to try

- turning down any request—personal or work-related—if it conflicts with a time already booked for your being active;
- saying no if invited to 5–6 P.M. happy hours you don't want to attend (if you're not ready for an outright no, then at least say you'll show up on the late side);
- saying no to staying past 5 at work unless it's absolutely critical.

If saying no feels foreign to you, it could be because you don't know the tone to strike. It's a challenge, whether the request is food-related or not. Here are tonal approaches[4], all healthy, respectful, and kind, that allow you to say no and thus safeguard your boundaries:

1. **VAGUE BUT EFFECTIVE.** "Thank you for asking, but that isn't going to work out for me."

2. **IT'S NOT PERSONAL.** "Thank you for asking, but I'm not giving to any charities until the end of next quarter."

3. **ASK ME LATER.** "I want to do that, but I'm not available until April. Will you ask me again then?"

4. **LET ME HOOK YOU UP.** "I can't do it, but I'll bet Chloe can. I'll ask her for you."

5. **KEEP TRYING.** "None of those dates work for me, but I would love to see you. Send me some more dates."

6. **TRY ME LAST MINUTE.** "I can't put anything else on my calendar this month, but I'd love to do that with you sometime. Will you call me right before you go again?"

7. **GRATITUDE.** "Thank you so much for your enthusiasm and support! I'm sorry I'm not able to help you at this time."

---

4. Courtesy of Christine Carter, Senior Fellow at the Greater Good Science Center

Getting Social Support in a Virtual World

Social distancing has shown us that you can feel connected to something bigger without necessarily sharing the same physical space. Some suggestions for nurturing support virtually:

Cast a wide net. Tap people far and wide who can best support your journey right now. For instance, if your sister-in-law who lives in another state loves to cook, perhaps you two could prep healthy Sunday meals over video together. Or join a virtual book club devoted to inspiring reads. Seek out those who can fuel your wellness journey.

Sweat in sync. Schedule a video call with a friend and stream a workout together. Research shows that people are more likely to stick with their fitness regimens when they perceive support from their closest contacts.

Create common goals. Set some intentions with your virtual squad to strengthen bonds and support your journey. Start with goals that feel attainable—a shared intention, say, to walk an extra ten minutes a day or begin the following morning with a brief mindfulness exercise. Then check in afterward: How did everyone do? Mutual experiences can help create a feeling of accountability and support, as well as enrich relationships.

Share, don't compare. Research suggests that passively absorbing the social media posts of others can spark envy and negatively affect mindset. Instead, pro-actively celebrate your network's triumphs—whether your friend's impressive workout or your brother's gourmet dinner. Their wins don't define or diminish your own. Then go ahead and share your successes, even just to post a selfie with a caption like, "Got off the couch for some fresh air and sunshine today!" Positive sentiment spreads through social networks.

Help someone. Few feelings surpass the satisfaction of doing good by helping someone else do well. Tutor, volunteer, pitch in. Find ways to share the expertise you inevitably possess in multiple areas. Those who teach end up learning and gaining more than those who simply wait to receive the lesson.

My Shift: Donald

A close buddy of mine, Jeff, happened to join WW and asked if I wanted to join, too. Jeff and I have known each other for years and went through similar struggles when we were younger. I was thankful for the opportunity to get healthy for our families together.

From the get-go, I found so much positivity on Connect; everyone really builds each other up. The hashtag #wwbros definitely spoke to me, enabling me to find guys who were working toward similar goals. At first I felt self-conscious about the idea of posting about my progress. Seeing other guys do it encouraged me to join in.

In August I reached my goal of losing 45 pounds. It's amazing that I joined with one "real life" friend and now have over 800 fellow members following my journey on Connect. Whatever path you're on, finding people who understand your goals and difficulties can make all the difference.

SKILL BUILDING FOR GETTING SUPPORT: THE TECHNIQUES

Close on Those Close to You

This technique empowers you to ask for support from your close relationships—people you see and spend time with regularly. Tone and details are key. The Define-Request-Follow-Up model breaks down support seeking so it feels less daunting.

1. **DEFINE.** Think of a person who has a lot of influence over what you do (someone you spend a lot of time with, someone you care a lot about) and

then think about what they could do to support you—the more specific, the better. Example: "It would be helpful if you didn't snack in front of me while we watch TV after dinner."

2. **REQUEST.** Talk to this person about exactly what you need, again being as detailed as possible. Discuss with the person how it will make things easier for you to reach your goals. Ask if you can return the favor, helping with something they're working on. So, if you'd like your partner to refrain from post-meal eating in front of you, provide specific details about the situation and what you'd like them to do instead: "This is really important to me and I really need your support. One thing I'm trying to stop doing is eating after dinner. When you and I are watching TV in the same room and you're eating, it's really difficult for me because it makes me want something, too. I was wondering if maybe you can go to the kitchen to have whatever you're going to have after dinner. That would be really helpful because I'd be less likely to eat something. Would you be willing to do that? And is there something I can do in return, to help you?" It's less a demand than a request. It lays the groundwork for why this behavior change would be helpful. It gives the helper a clear reason to engage.

At this point, one of two things is likely to happen:

    a. your supporter instantly understands and flawlessly executes your request, or (and more likely)

    b. some follow-up and fine-tuning will be needed.

3. **FOLLOW-UP/FEEDBACK.** As things unfold, let your supporter know how much you appreciate their help. Be specific about exactly what they did to help. This reinforces what they're doing and makes it more likely that they'll keep at it. Again, specifics: "Thank you for snacking in the kitchen rather than the TV room tonight after dinner. It makes it easier for me to stick to my goals."

If your person hasn't quite mastered the support you asked for, tweak it. You might say, "Last night, when you were eating ice cream in front of me, it was all I could think about. I was barely able to pay attention to the TV. I'm wondering if you could try what we talked about and eat in the kitchen, tonight."

Giving feedback in the moment can be tougher than if you wait a bit to formulate your words, but sooner is generally better than later.

Managing No

When people in your life ask you for something—whether it's to spend time with them, offer them support, or try a food they've prepared—you might often feel you must say yes because it's the "polite" thing to do. Sometimes, though, the things that are asked of you can get in the way of your goals. Saying no to these things is not impolite, unkind, or selfish—and can even benefit the relationship. When you're invited or asked to do things that conflict with your needs and goals, and a simple "No, thank you!" won't do, the following steps will help you to say no while protecting the relationship.

1. **DESCRIBE THE SITUATION WITH NEUTRAL LANGUAGE.** Be sure not to blame yourself or the other person. "I appreciate that you're offering me an extra slice of apple pie" is quite different from "You never consider my feelings and always push food on me when I don't want it!"

2. **ACKNOWLEDGE THE OTHER PERSON'S PERSPECTIVE.** For example, you know that the person is really proud of the apple pie she made and wants to make sure you enjoy it. You could say, "Your apple pie was so delicious" or "I'm so impressed you made that from scratch!"

3. **TELL THE PERSON WHY YOU'RE SAYING NO.** Clearly out-

line what you need—for example, "I don't want a second serving because I'm working on stopping when I feel satisfied" or "I enjoyed my first piece so much and I want to savor it. Having another will feel like too much."

──────────── ADDITIONAL RESOURCES ────────────

- TED Talk: William Clark, "Dare to Say 'No'"
- TED Talk: Chandra Story, "Social Support & Wellness"
- *The Seven Principles for Making Marriage Work: A Practical Guide from the Country's Foremost Relationship Expert* by John M. Gottman and Nan Silver

---

What's Next

Getting the support you deserve will make the journey easier and teach you skills that will enhance any relationship. It's also something to be grateful for. The next chapter shows you how to shift toward the practice of gratitude and find additional ways to be happier.

I CAN FEEL GOOD ~~ONCE I'VE LOST WEIGHT~~ NOW

Experiencing Happiness and Gratitude

You embarked on this journey to feel better. Happier. Yet if you're like many people, you think that losing weight or getting in better shape has to be an onerous journey, full of deprivation and angst. It's unlikely that you would describe the journey, particularly when it involves weight loss or maintenance, as a happy experience. It's no wonder people so often put off starting the process or get derailed at the first setback.

It's not going to be fun; this is going to stink. Screw it— I'll wait until Monday, or next week, or next month.

The effort is portrayed as drudgery by much of our culture, and by so many diet books, partly because the rules and goals are so stringent (see chapter 3) that it seems like awaiting a sentence to dieter's prison. It's also driven by the mistaken notion that any happiness or benefit can only be derived later, much later.

What if you could look at the journey itself as an opportunity to be happier? What if you don't need to wait until you reach some number on the scale to feel happier? What if you can feel happier during the process?

Happiness

For so many people who struggle with weight, the idea that you need to lose weight to be happier (or happy at all) is a dangerous myth, putting the cart before the horse. "Happiness comes with all these other benefits we don't think of," says Laurie Santos, Ph.D., Yale professor of psychology and teacher of Psychology and the Good Life, the most popular course in the university's history. "Some of the science shows that we have the causal arrow backwards. We think that if all these circumstances work out—you have a job, you're healthy, etc.—then you're happy. But research suggests that if you feel like you're flourishing, if you're in a positive mood, then all these other positive life outcomes, in a way, come for free. In the economic domain, we know that your cheerfulness at age eighteen, for example, will predict whether or not you have a job at age twenty-seven. It will predict whether you're happy with your job at twenty-seven. It even predicts your salary. We tend to think that high salary leads to happiness, but the causal arrow seems to go the other way." Of course, there are other elements influencing the job prospects and salary of a twenty-seven-year-old, especially in difficult economic times, an uncertain job market, and with structural inequities. But Santos points to evidence that everything from job performance to relationships and social life to immune function and lifespan can be predicted by happiness levels.

What does this mean? That the happier you can make yourself now—rather than waiting first to lose weight—the easier it is to engage in behaviors that help you lose weight. Yes, life can make it difficult, and you're busy and prioritize other responsibilities, and you might not even realize how much you've neglected to plan to do things that make you happier. But you can be happy *before* you lose weight. And, perhaps ironically, working to improve your happiness enhances the likelihood of weight-loss success. Happier people make healthier choices, such as eating healthier food, exercising more, and getting better sleep. Engaging in these healthier behaviors in turn brings you satisfaction, which contributes to happiness, a virtuous cycle that you can jump in on.

Who Controls Your Happiness?

One of the challenges to the notion of creating happiness is this common belief: We don't have much say in our own happiness.

That's what many people *believe*. When I speak to

groups or individual patients, I often ask, "What influences your happiness?"

Most people tend to guess some version of "life situation" or "the trappings"—their job, their partner, their other relationships, how much money they make, where they live, their level of education, the happiness level of their least happy child, and so on.

A smaller though still sizable group will guess genetics—"it's just how you're born."

Almost no one ever guesses that they themselves have a lot of say in their happiness. It's either the luck of the draw or the favorability of the environment. As in: If they awoke to find themselves in their dream home in their dream city with their dream job, *then* they'd be happy.

But we do have influence over a good portion of our happiness, regardless of birth, financial status, living situation, or a host of other determinants. Studies conducted by Sonja Lyubomirsky, Ph.D., professor of psychology at the University of California, Riverside, who has spent most of her career studying happiness, found that the portion of happiness that each person controls can reach as high as 40 percent. (Others claim that the number is somewhat lower, while acknowledging that it's in flux.)

It's crucial for people to *know* that they have agency over their happiness. One study found that when people understand that happiness can change, they're likelier to report greater levels of well-being and relationship and job satisfaction than those who believe that happiness is set in stone. In study after study, Lyubomirsky's research shows that there are things you can do to increase your happiness in ways that don't involve changing your circumstances. Small changes to how you think and what you do *can* make you happier!

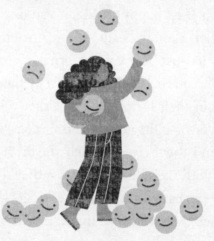

What is happiness anyway? It can mean a positive emotional state, where you frequently feel joy, pleasure, or contentment, which can be felt in the moment. Happiness can also be defined as life satisfaction.

Happiness is its own reward. "The intrinsic benefit is so obvious that the pursuit of it is included in our Declaration of Independence, along with life and liberty," points out Santos. Happiness is also a pathway to minimize the number and depth of the potholes you're going to encounter, because you've faced and triumphed over potholes before. You can get to happiness by doing for others, by random acts of kindness, by social connecting, by experiencing events or moments that elicit joy.

The happier you are, the less you experience stress, triggers, setbacks, or other negative feelings that lead to emotional eating. Is the key reason to be happy on a wellness journey to eat less or work out more? No. The number one reason to pursue happiness is because human beings prefer to be happy, enjoy being happy. Who doesn't want that?

Given that your happiness is more within your control than you may have believed, how can you increase it? Practicing gratitude is one way.

Gratitude

What is gratitude, and how does it differ from happiness?

Gratitude is a recognition of the good things in life, and being thankful for the small things that happen. Gratitude can be referred to as an attribute—"I'm a grateful person"—or as something you practice. It isn't simply the power of positive thinking but the constructive, uplifting power of realistic thinking. Gratitude enables you to find pleasure, even if it's in a small or seemingly routine thing (having a great cup of coffee, the night sky); gratitude shifts your perspective toward the bigger picture. When you hyperfocus on what's going wrong—which we humans often do—gratitude can help you lean into what's going well. If you tell yourself, *I can count so many things to be thankful for,* you have stated a fact. You have also shifted your mindset.

For example: It's a totally normal, pleasant day—or was, right up until you had a tense conversation with someone that really ticked you off. Thinking about it—and you can't help but think about it—clouds your whole day. Like many people, you're focused on what you want to change. You can't deny or ignore that something bad happened. But the negative mood dissipates if you choose to notice what's good in your life, particularly by looking at those everyday things. The practice of gratitude turns the focus on that negative conversation upside down. Now you're not looking for or obsessing over all the unpleasantness surrounding the conversation and its impact on you, but on other things, things that are right, pleasing, gratifying. You don't need to find a very big, good thing to remove the storm cloud hanging over your mood. (Yet another thing to be grateful for, since big things don't happen every day.) It's the small, often routinized things you're seeking. And since everyday things happen, well, every day, you have at your fingertips a huge supply of material to consider and feel grateful for:

I only snoozed the alarm six times instead of seven.

My yogurt and berries tasted particularly good.

I thought I was out of toothpaste but didn't realize I'd bought another tube.

I got a seat on the bus.

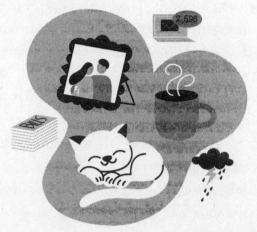

Do those feel too small? Gratitude is so accessible precisely because it's rooted in the available things in our lives. If you observe these things intentionally, your mind, after some practice, will naturally start to shift to noticing the small things with regularity, and to feel more appreciative of them. And they really start to not seem small. They are the things that make up your day, your life.

Of course, you can be grateful for bigger things—as long as they're still "everyday" things:

The sunrise is beautiful.

My family is more or less healthy.

I have a job.

> ### Benefits of Gratitude

Robert Emmons, Ph.D., psychologist, professor at the University of California, Davis, and one of the leading experts on gratitude, has stated that gratitude allows you to celebrate the present, to block toxic emotions (envy, resentment, regret, depression), to be more stress-resilient, and to strengthen social ties and self-worth. "You cannot feel envious and grateful at the same time," says Emmons. "Those are very different ways of relating to the world."

Regularly practicing gratitude leads to greater happiness—and, as stated earlier, happier people make healthier choices. Emmons, along with Michael McCullough, Ph.D., professor of psychology and director of the Evolution and Human Behavior Laboratory at the University of Miami, once conducted a study where participants were divided into three groups, each given a journal and different instructions: the first group was to write about whatever they wanted; the second, about the hassles of their day and what they wished had changed; and the third, about what they were grateful for from the day. Results showed that after nine weeks the third group was the happiest and most optimistic. The group that was asked to practice gratitude was also more physically active than the "hassle" group, reporting one and a half more hours per week of physical activity.

While the study focused on a small sample size for a relatively short period of time, larger studies have shown that being more grateful can benefit your journey—not only by making you happier but also by generating

- improved ability to respond to challenges and setbacks;
- improved body image (a more helpful body image is associated with an increased ability to lose and maintain weight; see chapter 5 for more on this);
- increased life satisfaction, optimism, hope, overall well-being, and mood;
- better sleep duration and quality;
- decreased levels of depression, anxiety, symptoms of illness, and stress;
- improved relationship satisfaction;
- greater feelings of connectedness and perceived social support.

One of the most profound benefits of gratitude is that it instills in you the belief that you can accomplish goals. And gratitude leads to happiness, and being happier helps you shift your mindset and can make the journey easier.

And, journey aside . . . who wouldn't like to be happier?

One of the challenges of a weight and wellness journey is that while so much of the work you put in has a long-term payoff, you may feel short-term rewards infrequently. You may be so busy focusing on what's going to help you lose weight in the future (e.g., healthy eating) that you pay less attention to what can help you feel good right now, while on the path. Do something healthy now, get your reward later. When you decide to have salmon instead of fettuccine Alfredo, it might not feel particularly amazing right then. If you decide to pass up a chocolate chip cookie, or you don't hit the snooze button for the treadmill workout: In that millisecond, it's not particularly reinforcing. You have to do some higher-order thinking. *Yes, I planned to do this workout three times a week, and this is one of those times. If I don't do it today, I have fewer days to make my goal, and I know tomorrow is unlikely.* Similarly, it takes some self-talk about why you choose *not* to have that cookie. There's no immediate pleasure in the decision.

Gratitude delivers immediate pleasure, by recalibrating your perspective. When you think about your day, the practice of gratitude helps you resurrect those pleasant moments, to savor them for a bit. Not for hours, not even for minutes, but a minute perhaps. It brings pleasure in the moment.

And the benefit in the moment isn't the only one. There's a lingering benefit afterward. One of the delights of gratitude is that it allows you to be less stressed and more positive about the *next* thing you do, whether it's having dinner with your kids or running an errand or going to work or falling asleep. By practicing gratitude, you go into the next event with a shifted mindset. For those on a journey whose goal is fairly far down the road, that's compelling. Do a gratitude exercise for five minutes or even just one and you'll feel good a minute from now, maybe five minutes from now, maybe a week from now. That's a pretty good return on investment in the short and medium term, while helping to buoy the long-term payoff. Oprah, who was ahead of her time in promoting the benefits of practicing gratitude, puts it this way: "Gratitude can transform any situation. It alters your vibration, moving you from negative energy to positive. It's the quickest, easiest, most powerful way to affect change in your life—this I know for sure."

And there's a further potential benefit to practicing gratitude: Research by professors of psychology Monica Bartlett, Ph.D., of Gonzaga University, and David DeSteno, Ph.D., of Northeastern University, suggests that gratitude, a "pro-social emotion," fuels you to want to help others, including donating to charity, engaging in sustainable practices, and more—and your future self is someone you want to do good things for, too. Do you decide to eat the second piece of cake now? Or does that "hurt" your future self, who wants to be a little healthier? Research shows that gratitude can help guide decisions that prioritize your future self.

Some general truths about gratitude to keep in mind:

Nothing is too small to warrant gratitude. When you begin practicing gratitude techniques, it may be difficult to look beyond the things that aren't going so well in your life. Recognize everyday events, like the smell of coffee in the morning, on top of the big things. The more often you practice noticing these moments, the more natural it will become.

Practicing gratitude is not meant only for tough times. Studies show that individuals may benefit from gratitude even during the most difficult times. However, this might be precisely the time when practicing gratitude is most challenging. Incorporate gratitude techniques into your regular routine. By doing them when things are going well, it'll be easier to use them when things aren't.

Turn gratitude into a routine. Once you choose one of the gratitude techniques at the back of this chapter, try practicing it at the same time every week. This helps you transform gratitude—and a focus on the bigger picture—into a habit.

The more specific your gratitude, the better. It helps to focus on as many details as possible when thinking about or writing down what you're grateful for. This will increase your appreciation for events and also keep gratitude practices feeling new and exciting. For example, instead of thinking, "I am grateful for my sister," you could think, "I am grateful for my sister because she forwarded me funny memes that really saved my day today," which will help you to focus better on the reasons behind your gratitude.

To find out your aptitude for gratitude, take a moment to answer the following questions. For each question select whether the statement is Mostly Like Me or Mostly Not Like Me.

I tend to focus on what's right about things rather than what's wrong.
__ Mostly Like Me   __ Mostly Not Like Me

I savor good moments as they're happening.
__ Mostly Like Me   __ Mostly Not Like Me

I am a "silver linings" kind of person.
__ Mostly Like Me   __ Mostly Not Like Me

I notice and appreciate the good things in my life.
__ Mostly Like Me   __ Mostly Not Like Me

When looking back over the day I focus more on the pleasant things than the distressing ones.
__ Mostly Like Me   __ Mostly Not Like Me

I let others know when they have done something that has impacted me positively.
__ Mostly Like Me   __ Mostly Not Like Me

I count my blessings for the things I have.
__ Mostly Like Me   __ Mostly Not Like Me

I notice small things in everyday events that I am thankful for.

__ Mostly Like Me   __ Mostly Not Like Me

If you answered Mostly Like Me on three or fewer items, that's a start. The techniques in this chapter are worth exploring.

If you answered Mostly Like Me four to six times, you have a head start on a gratitude practice. See if other techniques can help enhance your journey.

If you answered Mostly Like Me on seven or eight, you're a pro! Another thing to be grateful for!

Whatever your level of gratitude right now, you can enhance it; it's not simply something "you're born with." Just as happiness can be enhanced, so can gratitude.

Can Gratitude and Happiness *Really* Help Me Lose Weight?

Two answers: We don't yet know for sure . . . and probably.

Although we can't assert with certainty that gratitude and greater happiness directly lead to greater weight loss, two studies show that, after practicing gratitude, respondents expressed a more positive body image.

We do know this: Finding ways to feel happy and

shifting your mindset to a more grateful perspective create an emotional and psychological lift that tends to lead to healthier behaviors. It also turns upside down the premise that the journey has to be drudgery; that the more unpleasant, the better the results.

If you ask yourself, "Why am I on this journey?" the first, most obvious answer might be, "to lose weight." But most people don't want to lose weight just to lose weight. If pressed, you might say, "I want to lose weight because I want to be healthy." But that answer's not the full story either. There's a reason you want to be healthy. You feel better, you move around better, you want to be around for the kids and/or grandkids. *People want to lose weight because they want to feel better.*

You want to shift your mindset from "I'll feel better when I lose the weight" to "I want to help myself feel good regardless of how much I weigh." The techniques to come are designed to help you do this.

There's another way in which the weight-loss journey is often approached with an unhelpful mindset, making the road ahead seem uncertain and distasteful: *I need to leave my life to lose weight.* So many people think they must symbolically or literally "leave" their life and massively change behavior to lose weight: stop eating certain types of food, stop eating with the family, stop eating food they enjoy, stop being a night owl and start waking at 6 A.M. to get on the treadmill, and so on. "Leaving" keeps the door open to "returning" to their life and putting the weight right back on.

Does it have to be that way? Can the weight and wellness journey be integrated into your life, as part of a more holistic, inclusive version of who you are?

I know you probably came to this book to find a better way to lose weight or be healthier. You're in the last chapter, so I thank you for sticking with the ideas in here about mindset shift. My hope is that what you take away from this book is that you have the power to feel good and be happy, whether or not you have (yet) lost the ten or twenty or forty pounds you hoped to lose, or no weight at all. Here's the key: Your happiness is something you can influence, something separate from your weight-loss success. Our philosophy at WW is that when people join to become members, we never tell them how much weight they should lose. We don't tell them they *have* to lose weight to get to a better place or to attain success. Our purpose is to inspire healthy habits for real life. To help them get healthy in whatever way that looks like for them.

A WW member came up to speak with me after a workshop. "For the last three months I've been doing Three Good Things [one of the techniques in the next section] at dinner every night with my family," the woman said. "I can't tell you what it's done to our life, what the meals are like. You can't imagine how different dinner sounds and feels after each of us spends even just thirty seconds saying what we're grateful for."

Her words were so moving to me. She told me she had two adolescent kids, and how tough it used to be to get them to talk about what had happened in their day. (As a father of three now-twentysomethings, I understood the challenge of dinner conversation with teens.) The gratitude exercise helped her thirteen-year-old open up more, to become more grateful; he now actually practiced gratitude on his own. She said there were still arguments at the dinner table, still the occasional "spilled milk, literally." But the whole family dynamic had changed for the better.

Talk about a benefit that can't be measured on a scale.

As we talked more, she told me that the improvement in family life not only made her happier and more content, but practicing Three Good Things at dinner had opened her eyes to what was going well. She was able to adopt a perspective that made it easier for her to eat healthier, which made her feel happier. It was that two-way causal pathway, improvement in one area fueling improvement in the other. As Chief Scientific Officer of WW and a clinician, I was delighted to hear it. As a human being, I was even more delighted. The company's goal had broadened beyond only weight loss to healthy living and wellness in its many forms, and here was a great example. "Being more grateful helped me lose weight," she said, "but even when that wasn't going so well, I was grateful for other things—like my family and what I had accomplished that day instead of what I didn't. The payoff beyond the scale—wow. That was enormous."

My Shift: Krista

The things I've learned on the journey, though a lot of times they're related to food, I've been able to apply to other areas of my life. The concept of celebrating small wins and non-scale victories: I try and do that in the same way with my whole world. Maybe everything doesn't feel like rainbows and butterflies, but what's one good thing? What's one good thing that's going on or that I learned or did today? Reflecting on those things and taking more time to consider what's good has been a real positive, not just with weight loss but in navigating the pandemic as a whole.

It's not a structured practice. I don't journal. But I've incorporated gratitude more into my mindset—*What am I grateful for? What's going well?*—rather than the tendency to think, *Oh, things are so horrible right now*. Just shifting and thinking, *OK, but what's positive?* Some times are tougher than others but I take the things I learned during those times and apply them better than I did before.

It's just all the ways that it's benefited not just my weight but my mindset. The way I'm getting outside and moving my body in ways I wasn't before. It's been the whole package for me, and truly transformative. Yeah, I've lost weight. But there's so much more that's a part of my journey that I've come out of this with.

SKILL BUILDING FOR GRATITUDE AND HAPPINESS: THE TECHNIQUES

Make Time

Often we get busy and prioritize other responsibilities and might not even realize that we've neglected to intentionally plan to do things that make us happy. One clear way to increase happiness is simply to do more of what you enjoy.

1. **SET A GOAL TO PRIORITIZE AN ENJOYABLE ACTIVITY** this week, from one of the three categories below. Make your goal specific (see chapter 3 for STAR goal-setting)—considering what you'll do, when and where you'll do it, and who you'll do it with (if anyone):
   a. an activity you enjoy doing alone (e.g., painting, baking, taking a bath, reading);
   b. an activity you enjoy doing with others (e.g., dining out, going to a concert, playing cards);
   c. an activity you enjoy doing for your community (e.g., volunteering at the community center, going through old things to donate, tutoring).

2. **AFTER YOU COMPLETE THE ACTIVITY, REFLECT ON IT.** How did it make you feel? Happier? What thoughts and feelings stayed with you afterward?

3. **DECIDE WHEN YOU'LL PRIORITIZE ANOTHER ENJOYABLE ACTIVITY.** When it's time, repeat the steps above.

Awe Walk

Often we are awed by nature. This technique can instill in you a feeling that there's more to life than just yourself—that feeling you get when looking out at the ocean, at a beautiful tree, at the horizon, at the night sky. *I'm part of something way bigger.* There are other, larger influences in your life, in whatever way you choose to define them: the earth, the woods, nature, God, humanity.

Not only does this technique deliver the many benefits of physical activity (like improved ability to handle stress, sleep better, and manage weight) but it helps you to experience awe. Awe can increase our well-being and life satisfaction. And recognizing that there's something more than us can help provide perspective.

When people move outdoors they get a boost in self-esteem, energy, pleasure, and delight. They feel more inspired to walk again and to move compared to those who are active indoors.

1. **PICK A PART OF YOUR CITY, TOWN, OR LOCAL PARK THAT YOU HAVEN'T MUCH EXPLORED OR PAID ATTENTION TO BEFORE.** The place you pick might be somewhere new. It might be somewhere you visit often but on autopilot.

2. **MINIMIZE DISTRACTIONS.** If you're comfortable, silence your phone (or turn it off completely!) so you can tune in to your surroundings.

3. **START MOVING,** paying attention to your breathing, the feelings of your feet on the ground, the sights and sounds around you.

4. **AS YOU BEGIN TO NOTICE MORE OF YOUR ENVIRON-MENT, PAY ATTENTION** to what inspires or intrigues you. Do you prefer open spaces? Flowers? Old houses? Focus on the details. What do you like about these things? The colors? Shapes? Sizes?

Three Good Things

While I love every technique in this book, this is one of my personal favorites because it's so simple to do: You don't have to go anywhere, it doesn't take much time, and you can do it on a daily or at least frequent basis—and it makes you feel good right in the moment. Also, when you practice it regularly, you begin to seek out good things throughout your day. Take five minutes to follow the steps below.

1. **THINK ABOUT THREE GOOD THINGS THAT HAPPENED TO YOU TODAY.** They can be something common, like enjoying your morning cup of coffee; unexpected, like hearing a favorite song in the grocery store or getting a call from a friend; or something big, like going on vacation.

2. **WRITE THEM DOWN, DESCRIBING EACH IN AS MUCH DETAIL AS YOU CAN.** Document where each thing happened, what time of day, what you were

wearing, who you were with, and other details. This helps anchor the event or moment in your mind so that you almost start to relive it, feeling those moments again.

3. **NOTE HOW YOU FELT** as you experienced each of these three good things, and how you feel now as you remember them. Take a moment to savor these feelings; roll around in them for a moment.

Gratitude Letter/Email

When you're feeling thankful for another person, express it in a letter. This not only makes the person feel good; it enables you to experience the benefits of gratitude and of connecting with another person.

1. **THINK OF SOMEONE WHO DID OR SAID SOMETHING YOU'RE GRATEFUL FOR.**

2. **WRITE A LETTER, EMAIL, OR TEXT DESCRIBING WHAT THE PERSON DID OR SAID, AND ITS IMPACT ON YOU.** Be as detailed as possible. This is more than just saying thank you. Bring to life their thoughtful behavior and what effect it had on you.

3. **GIVE THE LETTER/PRINTED EMAIL TO THE PERSON AND WATCH THEM READ IT.** Research shows that this shared experience helps to instill good feelings in both individuals. And if you don't feel com-

fortable giving the letter directly to the other person, or you're not in a position to do so, send it to them by mail, email, or text.

ADDITIONAL RESOURCES

- *Gratitude Works!: A 21-Day Program for Creating Emotional Prosperity* by Robert Emmons
- *The Myths of Happiness: What Should Make You Happy, but Doesn't, What Shouldn't Make You Happy, but Does* by Sonja Lyubomirsky
- *What I Know for Sure* by Oprah Winfrey
- The Science of Happiness Podcast by Greater Good. Episode 1: "Three Good Things" and Episode 31: "Noticing the Good in Your Life."

Interested in learning more about WW? Scan the code for a special offer.

Final Thoughts

Mindset matters.

Changing what you eat and how you move is necessary for success in the long term—but it's not sufficient. True long-term change requires a fundamental shift in the way you think about the journey and yourself. I hope this book has helped to convince you of the benefits of these mindset shifts for the weight and wellness journey and beyond. I hope you've learned *how* to change your mindset, whether through practicing self-compassion, countering unhelpful thinking styles, setting goals and forming habits, leaning into your strengths, valuing your body as it is, finding your people, or experiencing happiness and gratitude. Some of these shifts will undoubtedly resonate more than others, and I encourage you to follow your instinct.

Just as changing your eating habits and activity habits takes time, so does changing your thinking habits. Be patient and remember self-compassion. Remember that your weight is not your worth; that you are worth taking care of no matter what you weigh; and that any weight-loss journey is best grounded in the belief of your own value, as is, today. Right now.

I wish you great success on your journey. And I'll say it one final time:

Be patient. Be kind to yourself.

ACKNOWLEDGMENTS

Writing this book has been a journey, for which I am extremely grateful, but it was not a solo endeavor. First, I would like to thank Andy Postman, without whom this book literally would not have been possible. Andy's exceptional writing skills, keen intellect, quick wit, and natural curiosity were extremely valuable and appreciated during this process.

I'd also like to thank my WW colleague, Megan Schreier. Megan, more than any other person, has helped establish a science-based fund of knowledge at WW as the mindset pillar of our program. Her behind-the-scenes, systematic, and scholarly work to cull the scientific literature for techniques that change behavior are leveraged throughout this book. I am also grateful to Megan for her multiple reads and helpful edits.

I'd like to thank the experts who made themselves available for conversations as I wrote this book. Being able to tap into their clinical and scientific expertise was a gift I genuinely appreciate. Specifically, I wish to thank Judy Beck, Gary Bennett, Deborah Busis, Amy Gorin, Neal Mayerson, Kristin Neff, Dianne Neumark-Sztainer, Rebecca Puhl, and Laurie Santos.

I'd also like to thank my various professional families throughout my career at the University of Pennsylvania, Temple University, and WW, all of whom have had a significant influence on my own thinking. From the beginning of my career, the mighty trio of Mickey Stunkard, Kelly Brownell, and Tom Wadden at Penn opened my eyes to the possibilities of impactful scholarship in an area that has been so misunderstood. In particular, Tom Wadden has been an exceptional friend and mentor. He taught me how to think and write about science and, more importantly, how to provide evidence-based and compassionate care.

I want to thank my WW family, particularly our CEO, Sima Sistani, who has enthusiastically supported *The Shift* and the principles behind it. One of the great things about working at WW is the depth and breadth of talent, compassion, and purpose across multiple areas of the organization. I want especially to thank Erin Quinlan for her multiple reads and helpful editing. I am extraordinarily grateful to Dawn Sobczak for her expert and kind assistance in every aspect of my professional life.

I would like to thank Jill Herzig for lighting the

initial fire that became this book, and Mel Berger at WME for his expert stewardship. Thanks to Karolin Schnoor for her eloquent illustrations.

I would like to thank Elizabeth Beier at St. Martin's Press, the talented, kind, unflappable executive editor; as well as Hannah Phillips and the whole team for expertly shepherding the book through its various iterations, making it better at every stop.

I'd like to thank the many patients I worked with at Penn and Temple, as well as the WW members who have invited me on their personal journeys. It's always an honor and a privilege when people share their most vulnerable moments. While I am grateful for the opportunity to facilitate shifts among the people with whom I've worked, I have always come away receiving much more than I gave. I want to particularly thank the WW members who shared their personal shifts in the book.

Finally, I want to thank the people who mean the most to me: my wife, Kathleen; and our children, Katie, Ryan, and Kevin. Each of them has been a great source of pleasure and pride since the moment I met them. Each of them, in their own way, has helped me shift my thinking in areas too numerous to mention. I am grateful for their support not only during the writing of this book but throughout my entire personal and professional life.

NOTES

Introduction: I'll Lose Weight by Changing the Way I ~~Eat~~ Think: Shifting Your Mindset

9 *A recent study using:* Tseng, J., and Poppenk, J. Brain meta-state transitions demarcate thoughts across task contexts exposing the mental noise of trait neuroticism. *Natural Communications,* 2020;11:Article 3480. doi.org/10.1038/s41467-020-17255-9.

Mindset Shift 1: I Must Be ~~Tough on~~ Kind to Myself to Lose Weight: Embracing Self-Compassion

20 *There are three crucial:* Neff, K. D. Self-compassion: An alternative conceptualization of a healthy attitude toward oneself. *Self and Identity,* 2003;2: 85–102.

22 *One study of women:* Adams, C. E., and Leary, M. R. Promoting self-compassionate attitudes toward eating among restrictive and guilty eaters. *Journal of Social and Clinical Psychology,* 2007;26:1120–1144.

22 *The self-compassion group:* Mantzios, M., and Wilson, J. C. Exploring mindfulness and mindfulness with self-compassion-centered interventions to assist weight loss: Theoretical considerations and preliminary results of a randomized pilot study. *Mindfulness,* 2015;6:824–835. doi.org/10.1007/s12671-014-0325-z

22 *Research on weight loss:* Thøgersen-Ntoumani, C., Dodos, L. A., Stenling, A., and Ntoumanis, N. Does self-compassion help to deal with dietary lapses

among overweight and obese adults who pursue weight-loss goals? *British Journal of Health Psychology*, 2020. doi.org/10.1111/bjhp.12499.

22 *likely because they're better:* Neff, Self-compassion.

23 *You're more likely to:* Sirois, F. M., et al. Self-compassion, stress, and coping in the context of chronic illness. *Self and Identity*, 2015;14(3):334–347; Terry, M. L., et al. Self-compassionate reactions to health threats. *Personality and Social Psychology Bulletin*, 2013;39(7):911–926.

23 *You're less stressed:* Neff, Self-compassion; Gilbert, P. (Ed.) *Compassion: Conceptualisations, Research, and Use in Psychotherapy*, Routledge, 2005; Leary, M. R., et al. Self-compassion and reactions to unpleasant self-relevant events: the implications of treating oneself kindly. *Journal of Personality and Social Psychology*, 2007;92:887–904.

23 *You're motivated to be:* Magnus, C. M. R., Kowalski, K. C., and McHugh, T. L. F. The role of self-compassion in women's self-determined motives to exercise and exercise-related outcomes. *Self and Identity*, 2010;9:363–382.

23 *You're better able to:* Neff, Self-compassion; Gilbert, *Compassion*; Leary et al., Self-compassion and reactions.

23 *You're less afraid of:* Prowse, E., Bore, M., and Dyer, S. Eating disorder symptomatology, body image, and mindfulness: Findings in a non-clinical sample. *Clinical Psychologist*, 2013;1:77–87.

23 *You have a generally:* Neff, Self-compassion; Gilbert, *Compassion*; Leary et al., Self-compassion and reactions.

23 *You have a better:* ibid.

27 *of these misguided beliefs:* Neff, K. D., and Dahm, K. A. Self-compassion: What it is, what it does, and how it relates to mindfulness. In M. Robinson, B. Meier and B. Ostrafin (Eds.), *Mindfulness and Self-Regulation* (pp. 121–140). Springer, 2014.

29 *The myth that self-criticism:* ibid.

34 *When you beat yourself:* Powers, Theodore A., Koestner, Richard, and Zuroff, David C. Self-criticism, goal motivation, and goal progress. *Journal of Social and Clinical Psychology*, 2007;26(7):826–840.

34 *Except that, as stated:* Neff and Dahm, Self-compassion: What it is.

35 *Approaching failure and difficulty:* Leary et al., Self-compassion and reactions; Neff and Dahm, Self-compassion: What it is.

36 *People who treat themselves:* Sirois et al., Self-compassion, stress; Terry et al., Self-compassionate reactions.

38 *Talk to Yourself Like a Friend:* Neff, K. D., and Germer, C. K. A pilot study and randomized controlled trial of the mindful self-compassion program. *Journal of Clinical Psychology,* 2013;69(1):28–44; How would you treat a friend? Greater Good in Action website. Accessed April 5, 2021. ggia.berkeley.edu /practice/how_would_you_treat_a_friend.

39 *Note to Self:* Self-compassionate letter. Greater Good in Action website. Accessed April 5, 2021. ggia.berkeley.edu/practice/self_compassionate_letter; Shapira, L. B., and Mongrain, M. The benefits of self-compassion and optimism exercises for individuals vulnerable to depression. *Journal of Positive Psychology,* 2010;5:377–389; Neff and Germer, A pilot study; Breines, J. G., and Chen, S. Self-compassion increases self-improvement motivation. *Personality and Social Psychology Bulletin,* 2012;18(9):1133–1143.

Mindset Shift 2: I See Setbacks As ~~Proof I've Blown It~~ Opportunities to Refocus: Building Helpful Thinking Styles

46 *Carol Dweck, Ph.D, the Stanford:* Dweck, C. S. *Mindset: The New Psychology of Success,* Random House, 2006.

48 *We know from cognitive:* Burns, D. D., *Feeling Good: The New Mood Therapy,* New American Library, 1980; Foster, G. D. Changing the way you think: A challenge for long-term weight control. *Weight Control Digest,* 1997;7:693; Beck, A. T. *Cognitive Therapies and the Emotional Disorders,* New American Library, 1976.

49 *Richard B. Stuart's groundbreaking work:* Stuart, R. B. Behavioral control of overeating. *Behaviour Research and Therapy,* 1967;5(4):357–365.

50 *More than two thousand:* ibid.

50 *Just as important, studies:* Beck, A. T., and Dozois, D. J. Cognitive therapy: Current status and future directions. *Annual Review of Medicine,* 2011;62:397–409.

53 *The good news is:* Burns, *Feeling Good;* Foster, Changing the way you think; Beck, *Cognitive Therapies.*

64 *Imagine you're throwing:* Stoddard, J. A. *The Big Book of ACT Metaphors:*

A Practitioner's Guide to Experiential Exercises and Metaphors in Acceptance and Commitment Therapy, New Harbinger Publications, 2014.

67 *Reality Check:* Foster, Changing the way you think; Beck, J. S. *The Beck DIET Solution: Weight loss workbook,* Oxmoor House, 2015.

68 *Noted, Accepted:* Burns, *Feeling Good;* Foster, Changing the way you think; Beck, *Cognitive Therapies;* Harris, R. *The Happiness Trap,* Trumpeter Books, 2008; Lillis, J., and Kendra, K. E. Acceptance and commitment therapy for weight control: Model, evidence and future directions. *Journal of Contextual Behavioral Science,* 2014;3(1):1–7; Jenkins, K. T., and Tapper, K. Resisting chocolate temptation using a brief mindfulness strategy. *British Journal of Health Psychology,* 2013;19(3).

Mindset Shift 3: I Should Take ~~Big~~ Small Steps for Big Results: Setting Goals and Forming Habits

72 *That's the crux of:* Skinner, B. F., "Superstition" in the pigeon. *Journal of Experimental Psychology,* 1948;38(2):168; Skinner, B. F., How to teach animals. *Scientific American,* 1951;185(6):26–29.

80 *Research has shown what:* Bovend'Eerdt, T. J., Botell, R. E., and Wade, D. T. Writing SMART rehabilitation goals and achieving goal attainment scaling: A practical guide. *Clinical Rehabilitation,* 2009;23(4):352–361. doi:10.1177/0269215508101741.

83 *Studies have shown that:* Wilson, K., Brookfield, D. Effect of goal setting on motivation and adherence in a six-week exercise program. *International Journal of Sport and Exercise Psychology,* 2009;7(1):89–100; Epton, T., Currie, S., and Armitage, C. J. Unique effects of setting goals on behavior change: Systematic review and meta-analysis. *Journal of Consulting and Clinical Psychology,* 2017;85(12):1182.

84 *A habit is a:* Armitage, C. J. Can the theory of planned behavior predict the maintenance of physical activity? *Health Psychology,* 2005;24:235–245. dx.doi. org/10.1037/0278–6133.24.3.235; Lally, P., van Jaarsveld, C. H. M., Potts, H. W. W., and Wardle, J. How are habits formed: Modelling habit formation in the real world. *European Journal of Social Psychology,* 2010;40:998–1009. dx.doi .org/10.1002/ejsp.674.

86 *When a behavior is:* Lally, P., and Gardner, B. Promoting habit formation. *Health Psychology Review,* 2013;7:S137–S158.

86 *New behaviors can develop:* Phelan S., Halfman T., Pinto A. M., and Fos-

ter, G. D. Behavioral and psychological strategies of long-term weight loss maintainers in a widely available weight management program. *Obesity.* 2020; 28(2):421–428; Jeffery, R., Drewnowski, A., Epstein, L., Stunkard, A., Wilson, G., Wing, R., and Hill, D. Long-term maintenance of weight loss: Current status. *Health Psychology,* 2000;19(1S):5–6.

87 *Research suggests that people:* Schumacher, L. M., Thomas, J. G., Raynor, H. A., Rhodes, R. E., O'Leary, K. C., et al. Relationship of consistency in timing of exercise performance and exercise levels among successful weight loss maintainers. *Obesity,* 2019;27(8):1285–1291.

87 *Another study found that:* Tappe, K., Tarves, E., Oltarzewski, J., and Frum, D. Habit formation among regular exercisers at fitness centers: An exploratory study. *Journal of Physical Activity and Health,* 2013;10:607–613.

87 *One of the truly:* Wood, W. *Good Habits, Bad Habits: The Science of Making Positive Changes That Stick,* Farrar, Straus and Giroux, 2019.

88 *One study demonstrated that:* Neal, D. T., Wood, W., Wu, M., and Kurlander, D. The pull of the past: When do habits persist despite conflict with motives? *Personality and Social Psychology Bulletin,* 2011;37:1428–1437. doi.org /10.1177/0146167211419863.

89 *True habits are slow:* Gardner, B., Lally, P., and Wardle, J. Making health habitual: The psychology of "habit formation" and general practice. *British Journal of General Practice,* 2012;62(605):664–666.

90 *Studies show that those:* Adriaanse, M. A., Kroese, F. M., Gillebaart, M., and De Ridder, D. T. Effortless inhibition: Habit mediates the relation between self-control and unhealthy snack consumption. *Frontiers in Psychology,* 2014;5:Article 444. doi.org/10.3389/fpsyg.2014.00444; Galla, B. M., and Duckworth, A. L. More than resisting temptation: Beneficial habits mediate the relationship between self-control and positive life outcomes. *Journal of Personality and Social Psychology,* 2015;109:508–525. doi.org/10.1037 /pspp0000026.

Mindset Shift 4: I Need to ~~Fix My Weaknesses~~ Enhance My Best Traits: Leaning into Your Strengths

100 *It's unfortunate that we:* Plys, E., and Desrichard, O. Associations between positive and negative affect and the way people perceive their health

goals. *Frontiers in Psychology*, 2020;11:334; Plemmons, S. A., and Weiss, H. M. Goals and affect. *New Developments in Goal Setting and Task Performance*, 2013;3:117–132.

101 *"Psychologists have learned over:* Seligman, M. E., and Csikszentmihalyi, M. Positive psychology: an introduction. *American Psychologist*, 2000:55(1):5–14.

101 *"We need negative experiences:* Reflecting on our strengths. Via Institute on Character website. viacharacter.org/topics/articles/research-points-two-main -reasons-focus-strengths; from Niemiec, R. M., and McGrath, R. E. *The Power of Character Strengths: Appreciate and Ignite Your Positive Personality* (pp. 18–19). Via Institute on Character, 2019.

102 *Positive psychology has shown:* Seligman, M. E., et al. Positive psychology progress. *American Psychologist*, 2005;60(5):410–421.

103 *Greater self-efficacy in:* Clark, M. M., Abrams, D. B., Niaura, R. S., Eaton, C. A., and Rossi, J. S. Self-efficacy in weight management. *Journal of Consulting and Clinical Psychology*, 1991;59(5):739.

104 *When people do recognize:* Seligman et al., Positive psychology progress.

104 *You can increase your:* ibid.

104 *Research shows that happier:* Boehm, J. K., and Kubzansky, L. D. The heart's content: The association between positive psychological well-being and cardiovascular health. *Psychological Bulletin*, 2012;138(4):655–691.

105 *The most extensive taxonomy:* Peterson, C., and Seligman, M. E. *Character Strengths and Virtues: A Handbook and Classification*, Oxford University Press, 2004.

111 *Research shows that you:* Seligman, M. E., et al. Positive psychology progress.

119 *Research shows that when:* Niemiec, R. M. *Character Strengths Interventions*. Hogrefe Publishing, 2017.

Mindset Shift 5: I Have to ~~Hate~~ Appreciate My Body to Lose Weight: Valuing Your Body

127 *And, as studies show:* Salci, L. E., and Ginis, K. A. Acute effects of exercise on women with pre-existing body image concerns: A test of potential mediators. *Psychology of Sport and Exercise*, 2017;31:113–122.

131 *For example, men have . . . degree of acculturation:* Sarwer, D. B., Thompson, J. K., and Cash, T. F. Body image and obesity in adulthood. *Psychiatric Clin-*

ics of North America, 2005 Mar;28(1):69–87, doi: 10.1016/j.psc.2004.09.002. PMID: 15733612.

130 *People who have overweight:* Cash, T. F., *The Body Image Workbook: An Eight-Step Program for Learning to Like Your Looks,* 2nd Ed., New Harbinger, 2008.

131 Sarwer D. B., Thompson J. K., and T. F. Cash. Body Image and Obesity in Adulthood. *Psychiatric Clinics of North America.* 2005. 28:69–87.

131 *Self-talk: how you:* Cash, *Body Image Workbook.*

134 *One of my first:* Foster, G. D., Wadden, T. A., and Makris, A. P. Primary care physicians' attitudes towards obesity and its treatment. *Obesity Research,* 2003;11(10):155–1274.

134 *Much more recently in:* Bailey-Davis L., Pinto, A. M., Hanna, D. J., Rethorst, C. D., Still, C. D., and Foster, G. D. Qualitative inquiry with primary care providers and specialists about adult weight management care and referrals (Under review).

135 *And they suffer:* Puhl, R. M., et al. Weight stigma as a predictor of distress and maladaptive eating behaviors during COVID-19: Longitudinal findings from the EAT study. *Annals of Behavioral Medicine,* 2020;54(10):738–746.

135 *While eating and activity:* Farooqi, I.S., and O'Rahilly. S. Recent advances in the genetics of severe childhood obesity. *Archives of Disease in Childhood,* 2000(July);83(1):31–4; Stunkard, A. J., Foch, T. T., and Hrubec, Z.; A twin study of human obesity. *JAMA,* 1986(July):4;256(1):51–4; Borjeson, M. The aetiology of obesity in children. *Acta Paediatr Scand,* 1976;65:279–87.

137 *In one of our:* Puhl, R. M., Lessard, L. M., Pearl, R. L., Himmelstein, M. S., Foster, G. D. (2021). International comparisons of weight stigma: Addressing a void in the field. *International Journal of Obesity.* https://doi.org/10.1038/s41366-021-00860-z

137 *It's not right to:* Obesity and overweight. Centers for Disease Control and Prevention website. Updated March 1, 2021. cdc.gov/nchs/fastats/obesity -overweight.htm.

137 *"What we see from:* Cruel Impact of Weight Stigma. World Food Policy Center website. wfpc.sanford.duke.edu/podcasts/cruel-impact-weight-stigma.

138 *A scan of anti-bullying:* Gay, Lesbian & Straight Education Network GLSEN (2015). From Statehouse to Schoolhouse: Anti-bullying policy efforts in U.S. States and School Districts. GLSEN website. https://www.glsen.org/research /statehouse-schoolhouse-state-and-school-district-anti-bullying-policies.

138 *Besieged by the critical:* Cash, *Body Image Workbook.*

141 *We know from our:* Pearl. R. L., Puhl, R. M., Himmelstein, M. S., Pinto, A. M., and Foster, G. D. Weight stigma and weight-related health: Associations of self-report measures among adults in weight management. *Annals of Behavioral Medicine,* 2020;54:904–914.

143 *We know this from:* Sarwer, D. B., and Steffen, K. J. Quality of life, body image and sexual functioning in bariatric surgery patients. *European Eating Disorders Review,* 2015;23(6):504–508; Matz, P. E., et al. Correlates of body image dissatisfaction among overweight women seeking weight loss. *Journal of Consulting and Clinical Psychology,* 2002;70(4):1040.

146 *A more positive body:* Palmeira, A. L., et al. Change in body image and psychological well-being during behavioral obesity treatment: Associations with weight loss and maintenance. *Body Image,* 2010;7(3):187–193; Carraça, E. V., et al. Body image change and improved eating self-regulation in a weight management intervention in women. *International Journal of Behavioral Nutrition and Physical Activity,* 2011;8:Article 75; Teixeira, P. T., et al. Successful behavior change in obesity interventions in adults: A systematic review of self-regulation mediators. *BMC Medicine,* 2015;13:Article 84.

146 *An improved body image:* Mond, J. M., et al. Obesity and impairment in psychosocial functioning in women: The mediating role of eating disorder features. *Obesity,* 2007;15(11):2769–2779. doi: 10.1038/oby.2007.329.

149 *What You Do for:* Cash, *Body Image Workbook*; Rosen, J. C. *Improving Body Image in Obesity.* In J. K. Thompson (Ed.), *Body Image, Eating Disorders, and Obesity* (pp. 425–440). American Psychological Association, 1996.

Mindset Shift 6: I Deserve to ~~Go It Alone~~ Get the Support I Need: Finding Your People

159 *What is known in:* Gorin, A. A., et al. Randomized controlled trial examining the ripple effect of a nationally available weight management program on untreated spouses. *Obesity,* 2018;26(3):499–504; Gorin, A., Wing, R., Fava, J., Jakicic, M., Jeffery, R., West, D., Brelje, K., and Dilillo, V., Look AHEAD Home Environment Research Group. Weight loss treatment influences untreated spouses and the home environment: Evidence of a ripple effect. *International Journal of Obesity,* 2008:32(11):1678–84. doi: 10.1038/ijo.2008.150. Epub 2008 Sep 2.

159 *more likely to engage:* Wills, T., and Ainette, M. G. Social networks and

social support. In *Handbook of Health Psychology* (p. 465). Psychology Press, 2012.

159 *less likely to regain:* Kayman, S., Bruvold, W., and Stern, J. S. Maintenance and relapse after weight loss in women: Behavioral aspects. *American Journal of Clinical Nutrition*, 1990;52(5):800–807.

159 *more likely to lose:* Kiernan, M., et al. Social support for healthy behaviors: Scale psychometrics and prediction of weight loss among women in a behavioral program. *Obesity*, 2012;20(4):756–764.

178 *Here are tonal approaches:* Carter, C. 21 ways to 'give good no.' greatergood .berkeley.edu/article/item/21_ways_to_give_good_no. 2014.

179 *Getting Social Support in:* Shanker, L. How virtual community can help you hit your wellness goals. WW's website. weightwatchers.com/us/blog/wellness /social-distancing-virtual-community.

179 *Research shows that people:* Darlow, S., and Xu, X. The influence of close others' exercise habits and perceived social support on exercise. *Psychology of Sport and Exercise*, 2011:12(5):575–578. doi:10.1016/j.psychsport.2011.04.004.

179 *Research suggests that passively:* Appel, H., Gerlach, A., and Crusius, J. The interplay between Facebook use, social comparison, envy, and depression. *Current Opinion in Psychology*, June 2016(9):44–49.

181 *Close on Those Close:* Brownell, K. D. *The Learn Program for Weight Management*, American Health Publishing, 2000.

Mindset Shift 7: I Can Feel Good ~~Once I've Lost Weight~~ Now: Experiencing Happiness and Gratitude

188 *But Santos points to:* (job performance) Diener, E., Nickerson, C., Lucas, R., and Sandvik, E. Dispositional affect and job outcomes. *Social Indicators Research*, 2002:59(3):229–259; (relationships) Harker, L., and Keltner, D. Expressions of positive emotion in women's college yearbook pictures and their relationship to personality and life outcomes across adulthood. *Journal of personality and social psychology*, 2001:80(1):112; (immune function) Cohen, S., Doyle, W., Turner, R., Alper, C., and Skoner, D. Emotional style and susceptibility to the common cold. *Psychosomatic medicine*, 2003:65(4):652–657; (lifespan) Danner, D., Snowdon, D., and Friesen, W. Positive emotions in early life and longevity: findings from the nun study. *Journal of personality and social psychology*, 2001:80(5): 804.

188 *choices, such as eating:* Boehm and Kubzansky. The heart's content.

189 *One study found that:* Van Tongeren, D. R., and Burnette, J. L. Do you believe happiness can change? An investigation of the relationship between happiness mindsets, well-being and satisfaction. *Journal of Positive Psychology,* 2016;13(2):101–109.

194 *You cannot feel envious:* Emmons, R. "Why Gratitude Is Good." Greater Good Magazine website. greatergood.berkeley.edu/article/item/why_gratitude _is_good.

194 *Regularly practicing gratitude leads:* Seligman, M. E., et al. Positive psychology progress: Empirical validation of interventions. *American Psychologist,* 2005;60(5):410–21.

194 *and, as stated earlier:* Boehm and Kubzansky. The heart's content.

194 *Results showed that after:* Emmons, R., and McCullough, M. Counting blessings versus burdens: An experimental investigation of gratitude and subjective well-being in daily life. *Journal of Personality and Social Psychology,* 2003;84(2):377–389.

195 *improved ability to respond:* Lambert, N. M., et al. A changed perspective: how gratitude can affect sense of coherence through positive reframing. *Journal of Positive Psychology,* 2009;4:461–470; Wood, A. M., Joseph, S., and Linley, P. A. Coping style as a psychological resource of grateful people. *Journal of Social and Clinical Psychology,* 2007;26(9):1076–1093.

195 *improved body image (a:* Wood, A. M., Froh, J. J., and Geraghty, A. W. Gratitude and well-being: a review and theoretical integration. *Clinical Psychology Review,* 2010;30(7):890–905. doi:10.1016/j.cpr.2010.03.005; Rash, J. A., Matsuba, M. K., Prkachin, K. M. Gratitude and well-being: Who benefits the most from a gratitude intervention? *Health and Well-Being,* 2011;3(3):350–369.

195 *increased life satisfaction . . . well-being:* Yoshimura, S. M., and Berzins, K. Grateful experiences and expressions: the role of gratitude expressions in the link between gratitude experiences and wellbeing. *Review of Communication,* 2017;17(2):106–118.

195 *increased life satisfaction . . . mood:* Lin, C. A higher-order gratitude uniquely predicts subjective well-being: incremental validity above the personality and a single gratitude. *Social Indicators Research,* 2014;119(2):909–924.

195 *better sleep duration:* Yoshimura, S. M., and Berzins, K. Grateful experiences and expressions; Wood, A. M., et al. Gratitude influences sleep through

the mechanism of pre-sleep cognitions. *Journal of Psychosomatic Research,* 2009;66(1):43–48.

195 *decreased levels of depression:* Wood, A. M., et al. The role of gratitude in the development of social support, stress, and depression: Two longitudinal studies. *Journal of Research in Personality,* 2008;42(4):854–871.

195 *improved relationship satisfaction:* Emmons, R. A. *Thanks! How Practicing Gratitude Can Make You Happier,* Houghton Mifflin, 2007.

195 *greater feelings of connectedness:* ibid.

195 *perceived social support:* Yoshimura and Berzins, Grateful experiences and expressions; Wood et al., The role of gratitude.

195 *One of the delights . . . stressed:* Wood et al., The role of gratitude.

196 *One of the delights . . . falling asleep:* Fredrickson, B. L. Gratitude, like other positive emotions, broadens and builds. *Psychology of Gratitude,* 2004; 26(145):166.

197 *Oprah, who was ahead:* Winfrey, Oprah. *What I Know For Sure.* Flatiron Books, 2014.

197 *Research by professors of:* Bartlett, M. Y., and DeSteno, D. Gratitude and prosocial behavior: Helping when it costs you. *Psychological Science,* 2006;17(4):319–25.

198 *Studies show that individuals:* Wood et al., The role of gratitude.

200 *two studies show that:* Wood, A. M., Froh, J. J., and Geraghty, A. W. Gratitude and well-being: a review and theoretical integration. *Clinical Psychology Review,* 2010; Nov;30(7):890-905. doi: 10.1016/j.cpr.2010.03.005. Epub 2010 Mar 20. PMID: 20451313.

205 *Make Time:* Peterson, C., Park, N., and Seligman, M. E. Orientations to happiness and life satisfaction: The full life versus the empty life. *Journal of Happiness Studies,* 2005;6(1):25–41.

207 *Not only does this:* Curioni, C. C., Lourenço, P. M. Long-term weight loss after diet and exercise: A systematic review. *International Journal of Obesity,* 2005;29(10):1168–1174; Jakicic, J. M. The role of physical activity in the prevention and treatment of body weight gain in adults. *Journal of Nutrition,* 2002;132(12):3826S–3829S; Pronk, N. P., and Wing, R. R. Physical activity and maintenance of weight loss. *Obesity Research,* 1994;2:587–599; Hill, J. O., and Wyatt, H. R. Role of physical activity in preventing and treating obesity. *Journal of Applied Physiology,* 2005;99(2):765–770; Coon, J. T., et al. Does participating in physical activity in outdoor natural environments have a greater effect

on physical and mental wellbeing than physical activity indoors? A systematic review. *Environmental Science and Technology*, 2011;45(5):1761–1772; Kerr, J., et al. Outdoor physical activity and self-rated health in older adults living in two regions of the U.S. *International Journal of Behavioral Nutrition and Physical Activity*, 2012;9:89.

209 *Research shows that this:* Peterson, C., Park, N., and Seligman, M. E. Orientations to happiness and life satisfaction: The full life versus the empty life. *Journal of Happiness Studies*, 2005;6(1):25–41.

207 *Awe can increase our:* Rudd, M., et al. Awe expands people's perception of time, alters decision making, and enhances well-being. *Association for Psychological Science*, 2012;23(10):1130–1136.

208 *Three Good Things:* Seligman, M. E., et al. Positive psychology progress: Empirical validation of interventions. *American Psychologist*, 2005;60(5):410.

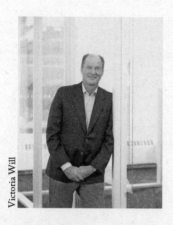

GARY FOSTER, Ph.D., is the Chief Scientific Officer at WW/WeightWatchers. He is the founder and former director of the Center for Obesity Research and Education at Temple University, and he served as clinical director of the Weight and Eating Disorders Program at the University of Pennsylvania School of Medicine. He is the author of numerous scientific publications on the psychology, causes, and treatment of obesity and has worked with thousands of people in group and individual settings. He lives in Philadelphia.